Brainy Babies

Dr Robin Fancourt, M.R.C.P. F.R.A.C.P. is a paediatrician with a special interest in young children, and those abused, neglected and disadvantaged. She has held several important positions, from President of DSAC (Doctors for Sexual Abuse Care) to founding and being the inaugural chairperson of Children's Agenda, a national organisation providing advocacy for children. She is also an executive member of the council for ISPCAN (International Society for the Prevention of Child Abuse and Neglect).

In 1995 she became interested in the relationship of the scientific evidence of brain development to the problems of maltreated and traumatised children, and travelled to the US to work with Professor Bruce Perry, a major contributor to the work on the scientific knowledge of brain development.

More recently Dr Fancourt has been central in the setting up of BrainWave, a national trust to disseminate information and lobby parliament for resources for early childhood.

To Professor Bruce Duncan Perry,
the person I am indebted to for both the inspiration and the
information in this field,
and
whose work, wisdom and generosity
has caused a revolution in the understanding of young children.

Brainy Babies

Dr Robin Fancourt
M.R.C.P. F.R.A.C.P.

Diane Ferrel.

PENGUIN BOOKS

PENGUIN BOOKS

Penguin Books (NZ) Ltd, cnr Airborne and Rosedale Roads, Albany,
Auckland 1310, New Zealand
Penguin Books Ltd, 27 Wrights Lane, London W8 5TZ, England
Penguin Putnam Inc, 375 Hudson Street, New York, NY 10014, United States
Penguin Books Australia Ltd, 487 Maroondah Highway,
Ringwood, Australia 3134
Penguin Books Canada Ltd, 10 Alcorn Avenue, Toronto,
Ontario, Canada M4V 3B2
Penguin Books (South Africa) Pty Ltd, 5 Watkins Street,
Denver Ext 4, 2094, South Africa
Penguin Books India (P) Ltd, 11, Community Centre, Panchsheel Park,
New Delhi 110 017, India
Penguin Books Ltd, Registered Offices: Harmondsworth, Middlesex, England

First published by Penguin Books (NZ) Ltd, 2000

1 3 5 7 9 10 8 6 4 2

Copyright © Robin Fancourt, 2000

The right of Robin Fancourt to be identified as the author of this work in terms of
section 96 of the Copyright Act 1994 is hereby asserted.

Designed by Mary Egan
Typeset by Egan-Reid Ltd, Auckland
Printed in Australia by Australian Print Group, Maryborough

All rights reserved. Without limiting the rights under copyright reserved above,
no part of this publication may be reproduced, stored in or introduced
into a retrieval system, or transmitted, in any form or by any means
(electronic, mechanical, photocopying, recording or otherwise), without
the prior written permission of both the copyright owner and
the above publisher of this book.

ISBN 0 14 0296921

CONTENTS

	Introduction	11
	Old knowledge and new insights	12
	The most crucial message	13
1	*The Centre of the Universe*	15
	The working units	20
	The driving force	21
	The ultimate control	23
2	*Wonderful Parents*	25
	The first gift	28
	The reception and recall of experiences	29
	One avenue: many aspects	31
	Attachment: the heart of humanity	32
	The special contribution of fathers	34
	A sense of belonging	34
	The rewards or the losses	35
	Maternal depression	36
	Other vulnerabilities	37
3	*The World Begins*	43
	The miracles of development	46
	The brain is different	46
	The power of the environment	50
	The specific effects of toxic substances	50

4	*Potential and Experiences*	57
	At birth	60
	The hidden changes	60
	Compensation	62
	Practice and use dependency	62
	Pruning	63
	The power of early experiences	65
	The sequence of brain development	66
	Other implications	68
	Timing	69
5	*Movement and Music*	73
	Movement before birth	76
	The working units – muscles and reflexes	77
	The tangled controls – the brain and the cord	78
	But not the monopoly	79
	The succession of motor skills	79
	Music, movement and creativity	80
6	*Mastering the Senses*	83
	Prime times	86
	From lullabies to language	87
	From seeing to vision	90
	Taste and smell	91
	Touch	93
	Pain	95
	Sexual feelings	96
7	*From Curiosity to Learning*	99
	The social and emotional context	102
	Flash cards, reading and computers	104
	Other avenues in early learning	106
	Reasoning and learning right from wrong	107
	The imprint on the brain	109
	Memory	110
	The multiplicity of memory	111
	The amazing memories of young children	112
	The loss of access to early memories	113
	The rewards	114

8	*Behaviour, Boundaries and Discipline*	117
	Behaviours and discipline	120
	When to intervene	122
	Positive and informing discipline	123
	Corporal and verbal punishment	124
	Boundaries and limits	126
9	*Sleeping and Dreaming*	129
	The basis of scientific knowledge	131
	The onset of sleep	132
	The patterns of sleep	133
	Dreams	135
10	*When Things go Wrong*	137
	Abuse, violence and a chaotic home life	140
	Early disadvantages	140
	The primary damage	141
	The associated behaviours	142
	Adaptive to maladaptive	143
	The impact of neglect	145
	Poverty and neglect	146
	The implications	147
11	*Nutrition, the Brain and Health*	151
	Before birth	153
	Milk: the first nutrition	154
	The influence of sensory experiences	155
	Poor nutrition	156
	The brain and physical health	157
	The brain and mental health	158
12	*Personality and Temperament*	163
	Changing the direction	166
	Negative and positive interactions	167
13	*The Challenge*	171
	The barriers	174
	What can be done	176

Appendix: New Concepts and Horizons 177
   Before birth 177
   The examination of brain cells and their connections 178
   CT scans 178
   Adding the measurement of function 179
   Functional Magnetic Resonance Imaging (FMRI) 179
   Positron Emission Tomography (PET) 180
   Electroencephalogram 180
   Event-Related Potential (ERP) 181
   Analysing chemicals 181
   Gene functioning 182

Glossary 183
References 187
Bibliography and Further Reading 191

ACKNOWLEDGEMENTS

To Tineke, Samuel and Nicholas for all they have taught me and to my husband Michael for his patience and assistance in the long hours spent preparing this book.

To numerous colleagues who have supported me, particularly those who share my passion for this information and have joined BrainWave, the national organisation with the objective of disseminating this material throughout the country in an effort to improve the lives of children. Dr Ian Hassall, Lesley Max, Judy Bailey, Sandra Edge, Jerome and Sophie Hartigan, Janet Lake and Professor Anne Smith are among them.

To Claire Hurst and Vicky Duncan for their assistance and guidance over many years.

My thanks to Penguin for providing this opportunity, especially to Bernice Beachman; to Fay Looney for taking many of the photographs, and to my sons Samuel, for the graphics, and Nicholas for the back cover portrait photograph.

Finally, my thanks to the wonderful children who have been my patients and whose lives have contributed so much to my knowledge and to this book.

INTRODUCTION

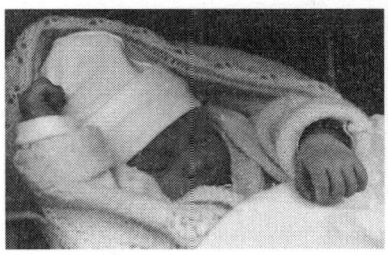

A new-born baby is cuddled and talked to; a father reads to his young daughter; a sister plays with her small brother. Unseen, a hidden miracle is at work. Instantly thousands of cells in these small children's growing brains respond. Immature cells are provoked to action, new connections are formed between them, and existing connections are strengthened . . .[1]

This book is about the development of the brain. It is intended for parents and others who care for and work with young children. It is based on recent scientific evidence about the way the brain functions and unfolds from conception to early childhood especially in the critical first three years. This poses both challenges and opportunities for parents and caregivers to ensure that the potential carried by the fertile minds of babies, infants and toddlers enriches their lives both as children and as adults.

As a paediatrician interested in how best to advise new parents and those who work with children, I am aware that the available answers have been incomplete. It has long been recognised that the way children are treated in their early years has a decisive and lasting influence. Many books on raising children share a central theme of fostering the quality of the relationship between children and their parents and caregivers. The findings of many studies from a range of disciplines have confirmed these observations and the need for strong attachments if children are to succeed.

What has been missing is the evidence of how these experiences direct and enhance the development of children. What are the crucial elements that mean one child becomes a caring, competent adult while another fails? The significant scientific knowledge that has emerged about brain development provides many of these answers and gives guidelines to explore others.

Old knowledge and new insights

The breakthrough for these stunning discoveries has been made by scientists and clinicians working in this field, as well as by increasing concerns for the well-being of children in this modern world.

We now know much more about brain cells and their connections as well as the chemicals and hormones used by the brain to develop and function. New techniques in imaging the brain display not only its structure and function in exquisite detail but how it uses energy and grows. Impressive gains in the understanding of what genes do and how they work have added to this explosion of knowledge.

Ironically, it has been the study of young children harmed by exposure to violence, abuse and neglect in early childhood that has added to the understanding of brain development and the needs of *all* children. It is based in part on studies on the impact of war on adults and the vulnerability of children to similar damage. Scars are seared into the brain by early negative experiences that fuel later behaviour. Research by professionals involved in child development and early intervention programmes for high-risk children have added other inter-locking components to this jigsaw.

Introduction

The most crucial message

We now know that it is the day-to-day experiences of babies, infants and toddlers that orchestrate the development of their brains. If infants are raised in a safe, nurturing environment, their brains will be stimulated by these experiences, which spark brain cells into action and wire the crucial connections between them. This is the process through which the experiences of children become translated into permanent changes in the physical structure of their brains. The critical timing for this occurs from conception to the age of six, with most progress being made in the first three years. What happens then helps shape the nature and extent of children's capacities both in childhood — and when they become adults.

Understanding brain development is to take an incredible journey. It is a journey into understanding the way very young children think, feel and react. It is a voyage of discovery that provides parents and caregivers with the scientific basis to enhance the lives of children.

It carries exciting challenges in how best to promote children's well-being and chances of success. Happily, what is needed is not any special or expensive equipment or endeavour. Talking, singing and reading to children, encouraging and endorsing their emerging skills, caressing, cuddling and playing with them are some of the ingredients required to build their brains. The power of these simple experiences can be seen in babies and infants who shine with an eager curiosity and a delight in life.

These are essential interactions for young children and result in the skills, knowledge and capacities necessary for a healthy and fulfilling life. In achieving this, these experiences must first alter the chemistry and structure of the forming brain. This avenue also brings a better understanding of the underlying determinants of different types of behaviour in children. The child who suddenly and with no apparent reason erupts with anger and defiance and is unable to be controlled, the child who is dreamy, disconnected and has difficulties in learning, the child who has problems in forming relationships with his or her peers can be helped with positive and beneficial approaches when the cause of their behaviour is known.

For parents, this information also sheds light on why their own abilities and emotional resources may be overwhelmed or absent. Why are some adults unable to bond with their children? One common barrier is lasting post-natal depression. We now know that such depression results in a reciprocal loss of activity in the infant's brain. This alone is impetus enough to provide swift, effective treatment and support for the mother.

There are many gains in understanding children and the profound importance of the first three years which comes from the understanding of brain development. To ignore this sound scientific evidence is to ignore the needs of small children knowing the consequences for many will be intolerable. I hope you will take this journey.

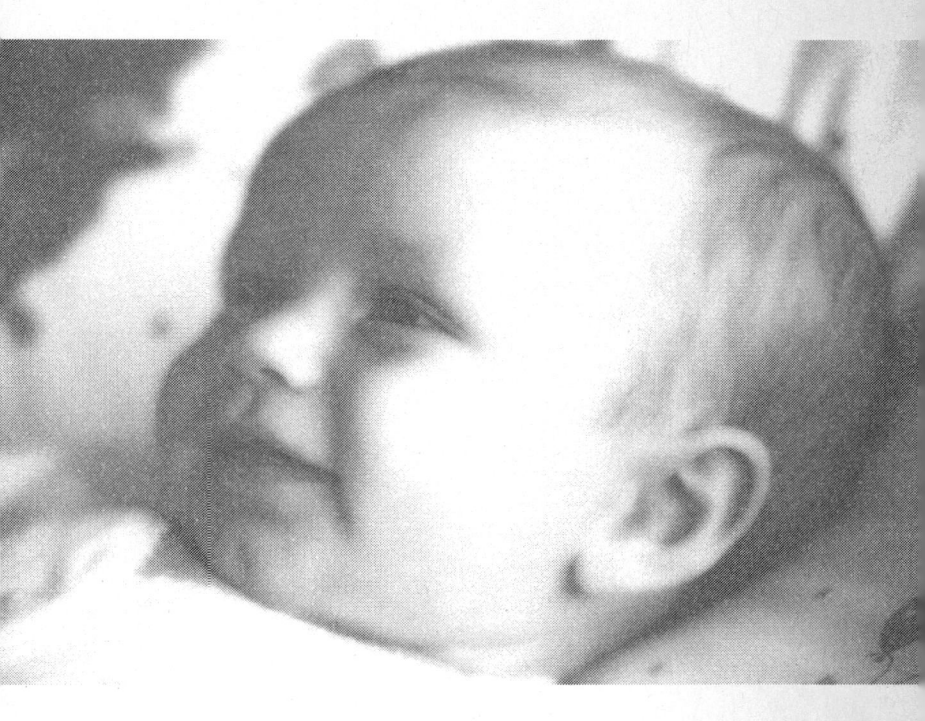

[1]

The Centre of the Universe

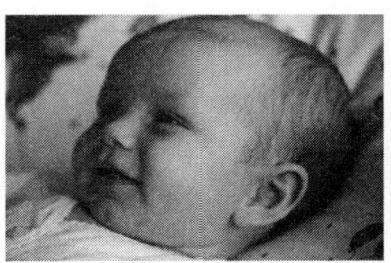

THE BRAIN is an unappealing mass of greyish pink wrinkled jelly. It looks incapable of anything. Yet what it does vastly surpasses any computer. It reaches beyond the control of such things as physical activity and the senses, to the opening of the mind, the body and the soul. It is the source of our humanity, our creativity, our imagination and our intellect.

The complex workings and the demands made of this amazing organ emphasise the astonishing requirements necessary for its development. It is the magic of genes and the experiences of the foetus and the child that control the development of this powerful organ. All children at birth, with the rare exceptions of those with inherited or metabolic disorders or severe injury affecting the brain, carry the potential to become competent adults when this development proceeds without disruption. However, a source of early damage in the womb can come from nicotine, alcohol or drugs.

A new-born baby cries. His mother changes his nappy and then cuddles him. Although his crying is, in part, a response from an area in his brain that unlike other areas is already mature at birth, it is also a specific response to his environment. The senses that drive this come from many different places. They may be in response to cold, touch or pain recorded and transmitted to his brain from his skin. They may be internal feelings like hunger and a need for comfort. At the beginning of life his brain is already extremely complex in its actions.

So what do we know of this extraordinary entity, the brain? It is made up of a series of organs and systems perceiving and sorting received information, swapping notes between themselves, and relaying information for higher processing and storage. Anatomically distinct, these organs are not independent but constitute an integrated system woven in a detailed tapestry.

Inspected from one side several of these organs are visible. An inconspicuous bump at the base of the brain is the brain-stem. This houses the networks governing the automatic reaction to stress or threat, often known as the 'freeze, flight or fight' response. It also controls all essential functions such as breathing, the heartbeat, body temperature and blood pressure.

The convoluted cerebellum can also be glimpsed. Working with other areas, it controls balance, co-ordination and movement, and may have a role in motor learning.

The two cerebral hemispheres integrate motor, sensory and higher mental functions. The left hemisphere is specialised for speech, writing, language and calculation. The right is wired for the ability to orientate its owner in space, face recognition in vision and some parts of music perception and production. These hemispheres are themselves divided into four sections: the occipital, the temporal, the parietal and the frontal lobes.

The outermost layer of cells, the cerebral cortex, is responsible for all forms of conscious experience such as perception, emotion, thought and planning.

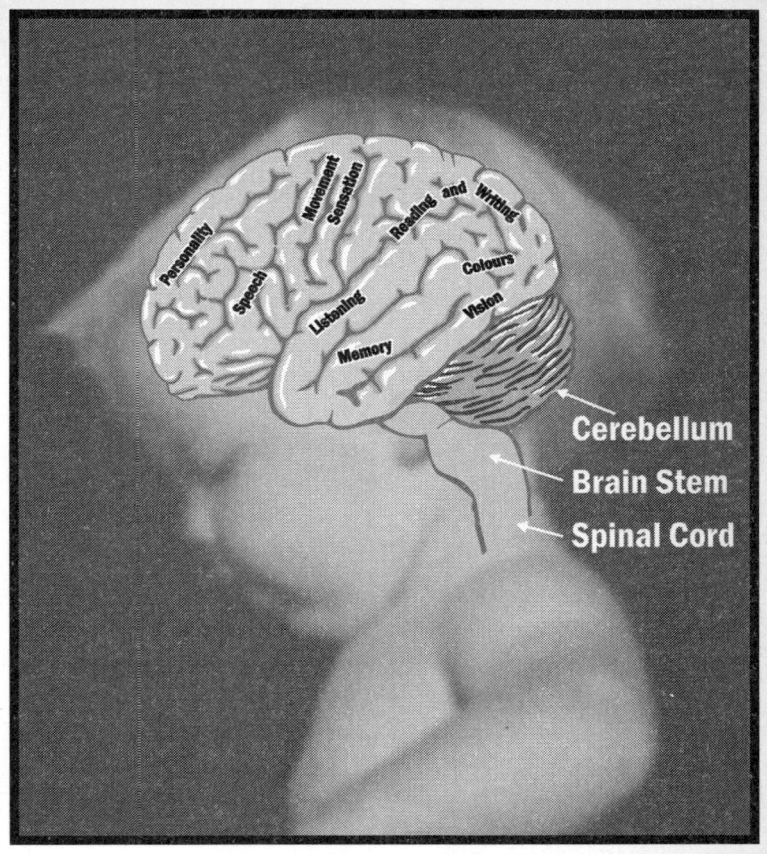

Side view of the brain.

The cortex of each of these lobes is furrowed with innumerable folds. These folds mature in a predictable sequence reflected in the progressive skills mastered by babies. So what parts of the cortex does the new-born baby use and when are other parts recruited? The baby's first needs are to explore and control his senses and to regulate his movements. As it is, those parts of the cortex responsible for this have already been in use before birth and will go on to develop further. Soon online is the temporal lobe, involved with hearing, language and visual perception. The parietal lobe is also active, allowing him to recognise objects and to develop hand-eye co-ordination. The frontal lobe, housing the networks for higher cognitive abilities such as reasoning and speech, will develop towards the end of his first year.

The other major parts shelter under the cerebral hemispheres. Their actions and their sequential development can be simplified if we view them in ascending regions. The lowest is the brain-stem. The next is the midbrain, which works with the brain-stem to mediate the state of arousal, appetite control, motor regulation and sleep. Next is the limbic system wrapped at the centre of the protective cortex. It is responsible for such vital functions as sexual behaviour, emotional reactivity, attachment and some of the processes essential to memory. The cerebral hemispheres complete this picture.

The development of the brain in the first year is amazing. It allows a new-born baby to rapidly achieve the use of his sight, hearing and other senses, as well as determining the shift from making sounds to forming words. It also determines when and how the baby begins to explore and to gradually learn about his world and about himself as a separate entity.

The working units

So what is working in the brain when the new-born baby cries, lies content, or watches his mother's face? The basic hardware consists of the brain cells, the neurons. They are designed to transmit information in the form of electrical signals to other parts of the brain. To do this each cell develops a long fibre, the axon, through which it passes these messages. Each also puts out a bundle of short hair-like tendrils through which it receives messages. Every brain cell forms connections with other cells, primarily by linking the axon carrying the messages to the input projections of the next cell.

These brain cells are not confined to humans but are shared with other species. The difference is in the number of the cells and in the number of connections. The fruit fly has 100,000 such cells, the mouse 5 million, and the monkey, man's closest relative, 10 billion cells. Each is equipped to live in their particular environment. In a restricted capacity that leaves many of these creatures locked in the present and forced to depend on instinct. The 100 billion brain cells humans possess allows planning, exploration, abstract thought, the projection into the future and the revisiting of the past. Incredibly — and unlike most other species — a significant proportion of the human brain develops and matures after birth.

The driving force

But there is still another component. When the electrical signal reaches the ends of the axons, they trigger the release of powerful chemical systems. Known as neurotransmitters, these chemicals assist the passage of the electrical signal across the gap between the connecting cells — like a spark in a spark plug. The chemicals themselves are manufactured in the axon tips, in tiny vesicles, like specialised bubbles. This process occurs mainly at night in sleep, with the amount produced available for use the next day. Not surprisingly, fasting, malnutrition and sleep deprivation can severely limit this production.

So if neurotransmitters are responsible for transmitting information between neurons, how are signals received from the body and how does the brain transmit its demands? How does it manage to control all the actions and interactions required to be human? To do this the brain must be constantly aware of all that is happening in the body and of all that is happening in the environment. To meet these overwhelming claims the brain must receive, process and respond to a continual flood of messages from millions of sensory receptors both within the body and on its surface.

The paths defining the journeys of these sensations are precise. Linked in nerves, those from the head and face travel directly to the

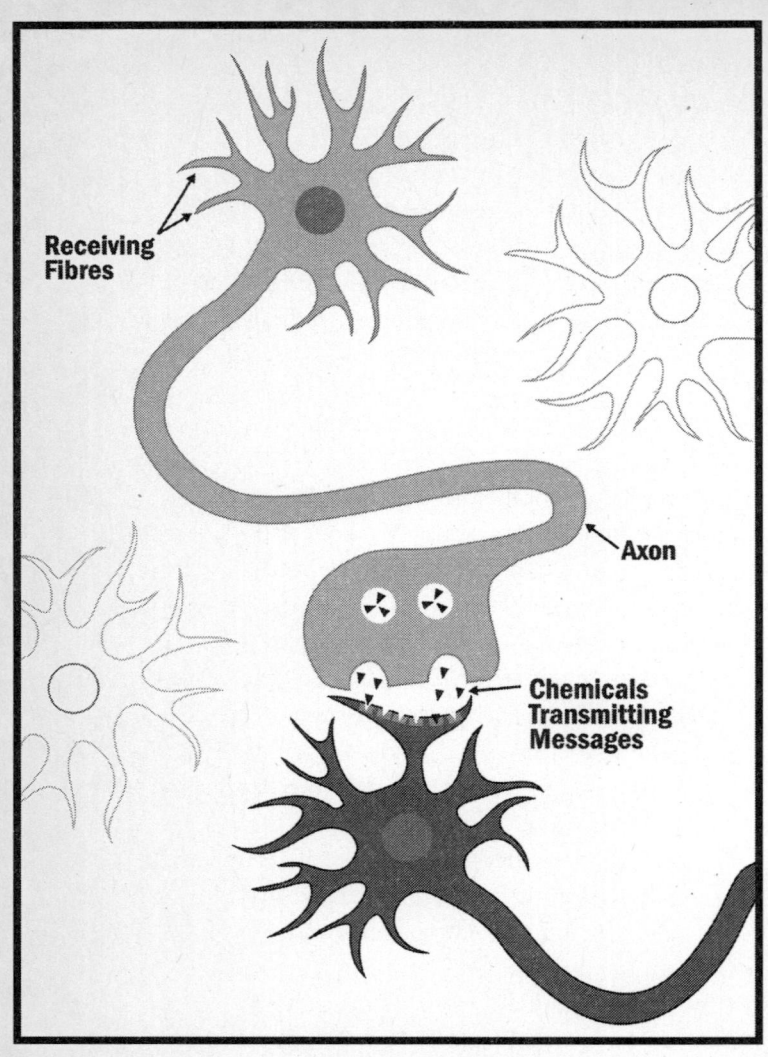

The connection of brain cells.

brain. Those from the body, the limbs and the internal organs must travel first through the spinal cord with each woven into intricate and defined ascending columns like a beautiful braid. Reaching the brain, the electrical messages are distributed to the specific areas designed to receive and process them. Once sorted, many are then relayed to higher regions to co-ordinate with others — to be perceived in greater depth, to join formed patterns of memories, and to contribute to any resulting command for action by the brain.

The brain conveys its orders using the same procedure either first, in descending columns in the cord, or directly through nerves carrying its messages. The nerves that are active conveying this information are known as the peripheral nervous system. The network connecting the brain to the internal organs is called the autonomic nervous system. This system has two parts — one to mobilise energy and resources in stress, and the other to conserve these in relaxed states.

How these extraordinary steps develop and so rarely go wrong is astounding. It's a miracle how a totally dependent baby becomes an active and assertive toddler in just two years. At birth, babies possess the basic form of all the brain organs, many already working but, like a paint-by-number design, there is much to be coloured in.

The ultimate control

Kim is a baby only several months old. Yet already she opens her hands and reaches for an object. It is not the tiny muscles of her fingers that have planned and controlled this process but her brain. As an older child she will learn to run and swerve to catch a ball. This impressive action links sensory, visual, auditory and motor messages as well as hand-eye co-ordination and knowledge of the impact of the ball to control its forces.

Just as the cerebral cortex brings the joy of Kim's first babble, it allows adults to indulge in imaginary journeys, to explore an extended sense of time. It controls our emotions, defines our psychological well-being, our sense of self, our spirituality, our values and a major part of our personality. Children raised by warm attentive parents in an enriched early environment have the opportunity to develop all these capacities and to contribute to life as they grow.

In early childhood there are the additional risks of deficits in or deflection of brain development through neglect, family chaos, violence and abuse. This brings a new understanding of the need for the prevention of harm to children in their early years and of the imperative need of early recognition and swift intervention for those who are hurt or troubled.

Fact file

- The brain is a complex series of organs, each with its own specific task and each interacting at a variety of levels with others.

- Messages to and from the brain are transmitted via electrical impulses. The working cells of the brain, the neurons, pass these electrical impulses down their specialised output fibres, axons, to be received by other brain cells through their input fibres.

- Neurotransmitters are complex systems of chemicals required to assist the passage of these impulses across the gap of the connection between the cells.

- The brain controls everything we perceive, feel, do and understand. It controls all our interactions with the environment and with others. It defines our well-being and is the ultimate determinant of who we are as individuals.

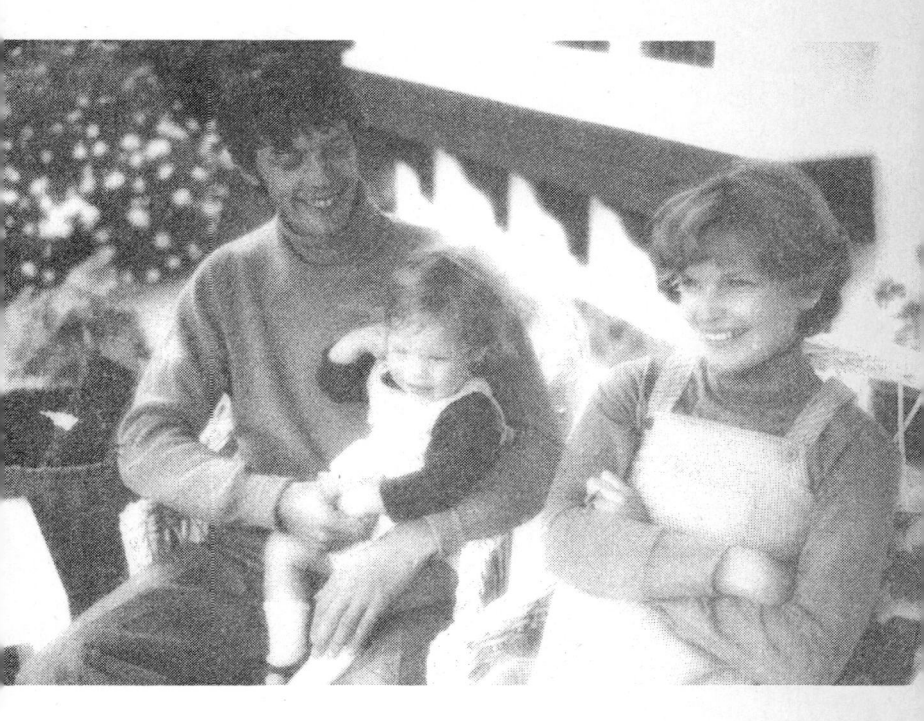

[2]

Wonderful Parents

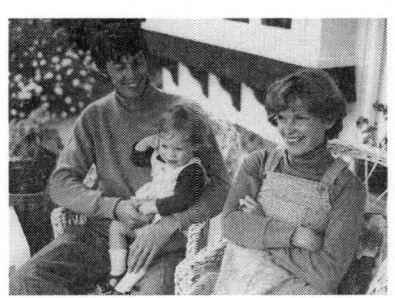

THE PAIN, triumph and excitement of a baby's birth is a miracle that never ceases to amaze and delight all involved. The baby is quickly inspected and is soon crying, announcing her arrival to the world and her own achievement. Later she is wrapped, warm and often too sleepy to suckle. What exactly is going on in her brain? Before the gifts bestowed by parents on their children can be understood, knowledge of the events involving the brain at birth is essential.

The challenge of birth is the supreme example of the firing and control of the survival or stress response. The brain cells and networks housed in the brain-stem are already mature. Catapulted from a world of warmth and security, the new-born baby is exposed to an explosion of new sensations: cold, light, touch, unusual sounds and a frightening ability to move. Such new experiences will be perceived as dangerous and an automatic survival response will be activated.

The neurotransmitters of the survival or stress response are a potent class of chemicals that include adrenaline and noradrenaline. Not surprisingly, the heart rate accelerates, respiration is sparked, and as independent life begins the baby is in a high state of arousal.

To counter this, the baby falls into a deep sleep when she is warm, swaddled and protected. This response is triggered by another set of chemicals released simultaneously with those causing the arousal. They are, however, not metabolised as rapidly as those of the adrenaline system, and include opioids, akin to morphine, that dampen fear and dismiss pain. The baby settles as her arousal abates, an all-familiar pattern of crying followed by sleep.

The first gift

From the time he was a baby, Eric was an infant who cried and became easily distressed. His mother was overwhelmed by these demands. Should she ignore his crying or continue to appease him? She was utterly confused over the profusion of conflicting advice on how to regulate or avoid regulating a baby's life. She wanted him to learn to cope independently but how do you go about this?

Most parents want their children to be able to deal with the stresses of daily life and recover from any devastating experience. Like Eric's mother, most parents do not know that the foundation of such resilience is determined by their first responses to their children as babies and infants.

New-born babies learn to cry to signal all their needs. The same surge of chemicals as the survival response comes into play. Leave him to cry so that he can control himself? The answer is no. Quick, consistent and, over time, repeated attention to a baby's cry builds in a flexible regulating capacity to future stress and, as the child grows, an ability to soothe himself. The chemical surge quickly subsides, the arousal is countered, and the survival response is modulated.

The foundation for resilience has been created for this child. Although this foundation will be compounded by many influences throughout his life and secured by a strong attachment to his parents, it is an invaluable capacity built into his brain at an early age. By contrast, babies who are left unconsoled or receive unpredictable responses remain hyperaroused, react more to other stimuli and can carry this set of problems into other avenues of their lives. They are at risk of remaining vulnerable to expected stress and to any major trauma.

A graphic example of this is found in research by Megan Gunnar at the University of Minnesota who has looked at children's reactions to stress using the measurement of cortisol, one of the hormones released when the survival response is activated.[1] One of her studies centred on the stress new-born babies experience when their nappies are changed. The findings showed that when a parent quickly and consistently attended to this need, the survival response — measured by the release of cortisol — was more quickly abated. These babies controlled this response in three months, unlike babies who received inconsistent care. Children treated in this way when they are distressed are most likely to become socially competent and secure. There are other important aspects of this research since persistently high levels of cortisol are known to interfere with the metabolism, the immune system and to have effects on the forming brain.

The reception and recall of experiences

Ben lies in his mother's arms two days after his birth. He is suckling, sleeping, crying, and has begun to look at his mother's face when feeding. How does he so rapidly grow from this to achieve mastery of his sight and hearing and an ability to move with purpose? How does his brain sort the swirling, unconnected, unlimited, surrounding experiences? What assists his learning?

As at all ages, Ben's experiences are received through thousands of internal and external sensory receptors. Those receptors on the surface of the body are used for such sensations as touch, taste and temperature. Their activation begins the amazing journey of electrical impulses that travel through selected channels in the spinal cord and in nerves to their ultimate destination in the brain.

Once these impulses have been received by the brain in adults, they are automatically passed down secure, powerful and permanent pathways. Ben, like all babies, does not yet have these highways and main trunklines. It is these pathways and their connections that his experiences are charged with forming. Transmitted, they are not attached to stored patterns of similar memories, which allow comparisons and bring explanations and solutions. These are the memories his experiences will create.

Ben's first memories are also different. They are not initially in the form we associate with memory, the memory that allows us to tell what has happened. These early memories are those laid down by all parts of the brain in relation to their function. Not surprisingly, they reflect the skills and abilities he is acquiring. They are visual memories, and memories of movement, touch, taste, smell and sound. They are memories associated with mastering the senses and skills that require no conscious thought. For Ben, this means how to cry, what taste is associated with what object, how to sit and later crawl. These memories are laid down throughout life in the same way, for example, as in learning to play a musical instrument or ride a bike, but never to the same extent as in these early years.

As Ben grows he is able to signal some of what has happened to him through his reactions. One significant event was being frightened by a puppy growling when it accompanied a neighbour to his home. In response he cries and attempts to hide when he sees any small dog again. This memory, as for all others in infancy, is recalled through the same sensations, actions and situations evoked by the original experience. Ben expresses such memories through his moods, behaviour, play and social interactions. At times Ben shows a regression in his achieved milestones as part of his response.

Ben's language skills will only be developed at two and a half to three years, yet he will clearly understand much of what is being said to him before then. Ben at four will be verbally fluent, but will still show his fear of dogs using his original reactions rather than by speaking. Significant prelinguistic memories are often recalled at a later age by using the original behaviours with a few accompanying words.[2]

One avenue: many aspects

Mothers quickly learn to respond to their baby's different signals in crying. That crying signal varies depending on whether the baby is cold, wet, hungry or in need of the reassurance of his mother's voice and the warmth of an embrace. Fathers rapidly become involved, and later, older siblings, other family members and friends. These lucky children are eventually surrounded by an orchestra of carers and admirers.

Incubated in care, they rapidly acquire an impressive array of skills and knowledge, and their active, busy minds display an understanding of infinitely more of their surroundings.

The time and attention needed by babies and toddlers is confirmed by science. The context of secure relationships is vital for learning; so too is reciprocating to a baby's signals essential to brain development. Just as practice is required to develop any skill or understanding, the interaction between babies and their caregivers defines the permanent pathways of the brain and the connections. In this unique way, these actions and reactions are the master architects of their brains.

One aspect of this knowledge comes from long-held observations of children and from the studies by the pioneers in child development, both without the benefit of the new technologies. Both confirm how critically important it is for parents to physically interact with their babies, as these actions are the translation of love and nurture required for brain development in these early years.

Mandy's parents and her older sisters have provided these physical responses. Mandy has flourished as a result. Now three, she is confident, engaging, affectionate and has an inexhaustible desire to learn. She responds to explanations and suggestions by her parents and is constantly asking questions.

Mandy's parents have never thought of the miracles they have opened. Their relationship with Mandy has endorsed and enhanced Mandy's every ability and all the knowledge she has acquired. Not just the skills but her eagerness to practise and advance in these achievements. The internal source of pleasure for Mandy is reinforced by the response of her parents, building her self-esteem. The safety of this partnership has allowed her as an infant to explore, to begin to communicate and to make contact with others. One thing above all, however, has won the prizes of early childhood. This has been the commitment of her mother and her father, a unique commitment seen in no other relationship in life. The prizes gained are an identity, a curiosity and a desire to learn, secure and enduring attachments, and resilience to expected stress.

Attachment: the heart of humanity

Jason is suddenly behaving badly at his pre-school. Tamara unexpectedly refuses to go to her grandmother's house. Crystal has stopped eating what was her favourite food and is arguing about going to bed. The parents of these children analyse what has been going on, and seek an explanation that will allow them to guide their children through their trouble. What is behind this response is their unparalleled attachment to their children.

This attachment and empathy with others is also at the heart of children's needs. It is the most important of all capacities they must acquire. It is essential for their enjoyment of life and for their future intimate relationships. It influences their learning and determines what sort of parents and partners they will be. It acts as a powerful protection in the face of emotional harm or abuse, adding to the initial basis of their resilience.

Like all other capacities, attachment is developed, mediated and organised by the brain. The effects, which begin with a mother's warm responsive attention, change the chemistry and the structure of the baby's forming brain. The architecture and the eventual function of the areas in the brain involved, like others, are developed in a two-way process between the child and the responses of the parents.

This responsive caregiving goes beyond physical needs for warmth and food to mediating the contact of babies and infants with the environment and adapting to their moods and preferences. The ingredients are things we take for granted. Nothing seemingly special, they are such things as holding, rocking, singing to, encouraging and praising a child with the quantity of these interactions crucial. Of all this flood of sensory experiences, positive physical touch is the most vital.

These experiences for babies and infants build in the networks for attachment and two other vital areas in their brains. One brings the sense of reward and pleasure that come with attachment. Having friends, belonging to a family, being close to parents, *feels good*. Missing this can cause devastating problems. Equally significant are the other circuits that are created. Those bring an understanding of the needs and emotions of others. This empathy, as with attachment, is essential to life in a family and the safety of the wider community.

The first year of life is the most critical in a child's ability to form attachments. The responses are modified and change as children grow but they retain this essential core. The physical nurturing begins with the mother but babies and infants are open to become attached to anyone who is consistently available and caring. These are fortunate children. They have the extra love and protection of their fathers, an extended family, their grandparents, and neighbours or family friends. The additional experiences and opportunities strengthen their attachments and expand their learning. Going to the supermarket with a patient grandmother who answers every question can be much more exciting and informative than going with a hurried mother.

Studies of young children in well-run day-care centres, crèches or kindergartens with well-trained, skilled staff and a limited ratio of children to adults confirm this evidence. The relationship and the attachment of children to their care providers does not weaken the bonds with their parents and for many, not surprisingly, enhances their cognitive and verbal abilities.

The special contribution of fathers

Sally's mother stays close to her as she explores the garden. Her mother is reassuring and protective. Sally's father is quite the opposite. When he comes home he picks his infant daughter up and sits her around his neck. Grasping his hair, Sally squeals with delight. He runs with her, pulls her off and throws her into the air. Gasping for breath, Sally demands more.

These different reactions are almost universal. They transcend social class and the expectations of many cultures. Fathers are more challenging, more physical in their interactions, and more willing to let their children out of their sight before going to the rescue. They will allow their children to explore independently before they intervene. In a potentially frightening situation for the child, they tend to stand back while mothers move closer. Babies recognise this as early as six weeks when they will respond to the sight of their mother by becoming calm, while becoming more active and aroused in the presence of their father.

These different interactions add different dimensions to Sally's attachment, to her emotional growth and her eventual independence. The father's active involvement also has other benefits. These children tend to have a better impulse control, are less likely to become violent, and have better social skills.

A sense of belonging

Equally essential is a sense of belonging — belonging to the immediate family, to the history of the family, and over time to the cultural group and community in which children grow. While this begins with a secure relationship with their parents it is added to in a multitude of different ways: stories of their own childhood, of their parents' lives as children, of family photographs and much-repeated family stories.

For lucky children it is the grandparents or other close relatives who bring the vital extension to this sense of belonging. They are able to tell much-loved stories of their own parents when they were little. They themselves grew up in that world full of mystery. They know things no one else does. They are at once oral historians, mentors and at times caregivers themselves. A strong emotional attachment between grandparents and children is second only to that of the parents. Other close members of the extended family, old family friends or neighbours can also assume this role.

The sense of belonging is built into the brain and with it a foundation of security that serves children well when the time comes to face the wider world with all its troubles.

The rewards or the losses

Early attachment becomes the template for all future intimate relationships. Being able to understand and appreciate the feelings and needs of others ensures that children can fully participate in life. A sense of belonging confirms their place in our world. Children who are left without this enrichment, left bereft of knowing where they belong, can remain vulnerable in later life. Such vulnerability is commonly increased by other experiences.

Ian is a boy left to struggle alone in this way. Raised in the crossfire of family violence, he failed to develop strong attachments to his parents and experiences none of the sense of pleasure and reward such attachment brings. With no sense of belonging and unable to learn the rules of social interaction, he has failed to be accepted at school. Now 13, he is seeking to fill the loss of his inner pleasure with highs through glue sniffing, drugs and prescription pills. His poor prospects are being further destroyed.

This story is repeated far too often — a failure to learn, to make relationships with peers, being left unattended after school or being isolated from any support by family or friends. As a society we are becoming increasingly isolated with television, computer games and the internet now substituting social interaction. Violent content of films and television can harden any developing aggressive tendencies and escalates the emotional damage of violence witnessed at home. Such experiences can lead to a dangerous sense of alienation that will grow and erupt in an array of other later problems.

Maternal depression

Mothers can sometimes have difficulties responding to the cues of their babies. One of the most frequent causes of this is maternal depression.

A mother struggles to respond to her baby's crying. She knows what she should do but there is an ill-defined dark weight pressing on her, a heavy greyness that blunts her motivation and any enjoyment of her child. With no words to describe what she feels, she does not ask for help. Unnoticed by others, her post-partum depression lingers to the detriment of herself and her child.

Without willing it to be so, she expresses little positive emotion to him, is not attentive, often fails to respond to his needs, and when she does she tends to be controlling and intrusive. The baby in turn becomes more withdrawn, less active, shows less eagerness to master new tasks, sleeps more often, and increasingly loses interest in his surroundings.

The frequency and consistency of the warmth and the nurturing this baby requires is diminished. The pathways and the connections open to change in his brain are not stimulated or secured. The measured evidence is seen in a rise in his cortisol levels, an accelerated heart rate and a reduction in the activity of area of his brain which is associated with outwardly expressed emotions such as joy, anger and interest.

If the mother's depression is treated or goes into remission before the baby is six months old, there will be a corresponding improvement in the baby. He will be alert more often, cry less, have lower cortisol levels, better sleeping patterns, greater weight gain and his emotions and social capabilities will improve.

If a mother's depression lasts longer than six months, the child may be cognitively impaired and display disordered attachment to his mother and, later, behavioural problems.

It is important that fathers, family members, friends and health care workers are aware of the dangers, and can offer their care and arrange for help. Fathers often buffer some of the baby's withdrawal with their stimulation and arousal of the child. Other forms of help, with excellent effects, have come through music and massage therapy for the babies and their mothers.

Other vulnerabilities

Other problems in responding to young children arise because the skills and the emotional capacity of parents to raise their children successfully are not inherited. These skills are mediated, developed and organised by the brain in early life and are based on parents' own upbringing. The abilities necessary to respond to children are available to adults whose early childhood was supportive, safe and nurturing.

Parents may lack these skills to varying degrees. Most inadequacies are minor but can be exaggerated in any stressful situation in the home or with the child. If a parent is facing escalating difficulties, they should ask others for advice and seek help. A trusted friend, a family member, a doctor or community worker may be able to listen and assist. Feeling guilty about asking someone for help should never be a barrier. Help given is a wonderful gift that can be passed on later with real understanding to another person in similar difficulties. Even when the required abilities and responses are impaired, many can be retaught successfully for the parent and child. As in depression, the soothing touch of massage (a simple example) can reward the mother and her unsettled baby, and alter their relationship.

At the most concerning end of this continuum are parents who simply cannot respond in any appropriate way to their young children. Neglect, abuse or a chaotic family life has marred their own early childhood. Emotionally empty, with scarred attachments and the absence of any related sense of pleasure, they seek their highs, like Ian, through drugs, alcohol or self-inflicted harm. Some are simply too young. Teenagers, whose own needs are unfulfilled, do not have the capacity to deal with the constant requirements of a demanding baby. These parents require early recognition and assistance. For some this may be through personal support and guidance. For others, programmes that have been developed overseas to do this have been successful and are proving cost effective. Some require statutory intervention to assess what is happening to their children.

Sometimes parents with every potential to be successful are simply overwhelmed. A child may be irritable, constantly waking at night and failing to react to close contact with her mother or father. Tired and worried, without intervention, a very negative cycle begins. When this happens, parents with every ability to raise children may not be able to rise above the challenge. Solo parents can be in the same situation when their personal and financial capacities are destroyed by the many disadvantages their situation can bring.

Fact file

- The way parents respond to their baby or infant will largely shape the child's developing skills and knowledge. A nurturing environment will allow the child to develop secure attachments, self-esteem, a sense of belonging, and an eagerness to learn.

Wonderful Parents

- The initial memories of babies and infants are those that build abilities that require no conscious thought and reflect the skills the child is acquiring.

- The foundation of an individual's resilience to stress in life is found in the nurturing, warm responses of that individual's parents during early childhood.

- Attachment and empathy with others are built into the brain through a flood of sensory experiences with positive physical touch being the most important, and the first year of life the most crucial in timing.

- The best way of raising secure children is to provide a secure family environment in which children feel they belong and that they are loved.

- Sensitive, responsive, secure caregiving plays an important role in buffering or blocking the effects of persistent negative or traumatic experiences in young children.

- There are many ways in which a positive relationship between young children and their parents can be disrupted — maternal depression, stress, the collective effects of poverty, and the multiple disadvantages that can accompany sole-parent households are some of the most common.

Things to do

For parents

- Parents are not responsible for providing all the necessary experiences of young children. Other adults and their siblings are essential for expanding children's skills, their relationships and their understanding of others.

- Remember that consistently responding to babies crying will not 'spoil' them but will encourage the babies to develop their own strategies to protect themselves and respond to stress.

- Focus on the time, attention and the ways you can nurture and endorse your children when you are with them. When you cannot do this personally, ensure that a family member, friend or caregiver knows about child development and can provide for their needs.

- Show children your family photographs and tell them old family stories. Encourage any grandparents or other relatives to do the same. The sense of where they come from and of being part of the family history helps develop a sense of belonging.

- If you are facing problems, ask for help. Similarly, assist other parents having difficulty in responding to their babies and small children. It is only by reaching out that this vital link can be secured for some parents.

- Remember that any unexpected regression in infants' and toddlers' abilities or in changes in their moods, play and behaviour may signal some distress in their lives. Although this can be minor, you should still determine what the cause is so that you can guide the child through the perceived harm. Major problems may require professional intervention. Be careful not to label these changes in terms of the behaviour, or treat them merely as a passing developmental stage.

For workers providing services to young children and families

- Parents' most important gifts to their children are time and their own emotional and financial resources. Their contribution to the community in raising children is a challenging and poorly supported task. Whenever possible, be their advocates and lobby on their behalf.

- The government will not act until the public demands it. The changes for parents and their children must start with community endeavours.

- Some local companies and corporations may help with funding. Usually some reward in promoting their business is a required part of the contract.

- In lobbying local or national government, set goals and progress towards these in a flexible way. Expect to make compromises before you reach your goals.

- When determining what your most urgent objectives are, ask local families and examine the requirements of local children.

- If you are lobbying the government or local council, join forces with other organisations with similar concerns for children.

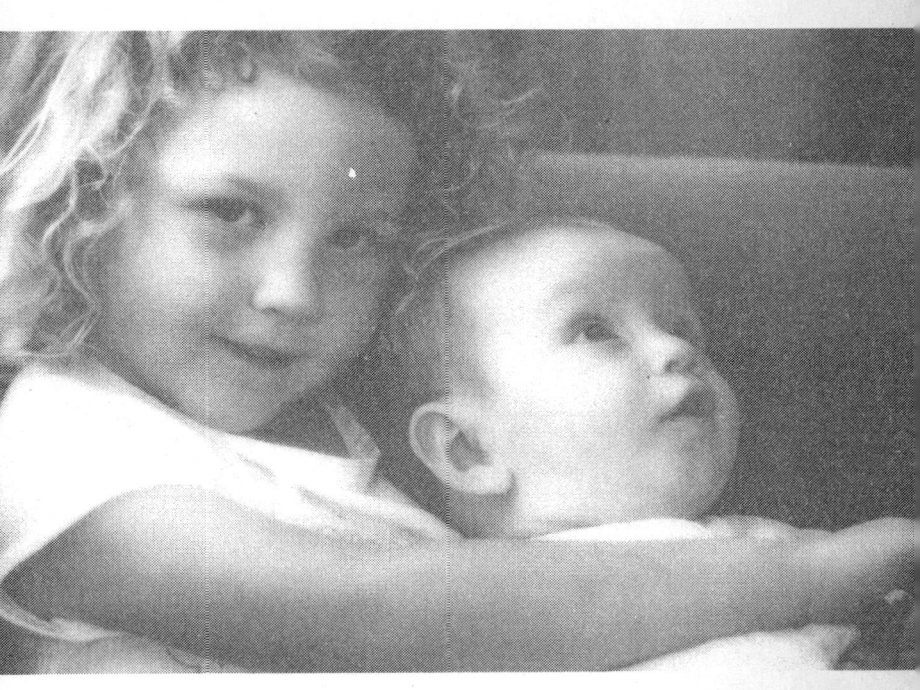

[3]

The World Begins

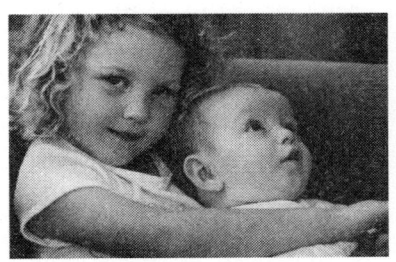

BOTH PARENTS show their joy at the birth of their long-awaited child. Their joy is, in part, the excitement of welcoming the baby into the world — a baby they have discussed and speculated about for many months. They touch her, kiss her, smell the distinct smell of a baby just born and begin to imagine whom she resembles most. It is a joy that also comes from the fact that the examining doctor has told them that their daughter has no abnormalities.

The hope that an unborn baby will be healthy is universal. Most parents know little of the extraordinary process of how a baby is formed and develops. Most parents know even less about the development of the brain. Just 15 years ago scientists believed that the brain before birth was passively formed and entirely genetically directed. In those 15 years extraordinary advances have been made. We now know that even before birth the brain is alive with astonishing activity dedicated to its creation with genes and the environment influencing its development. This spectacular display opens the horizons for the incredible and rapid learning of the new-born child. The intertwined steps dismiss the long-held arguments over the influences of nature or nurture in showing that the brain develops as an interplay between the two, even before birth.

The miracles of development

There is so much that is almost beyond comprehension in the creation of a baby from a single fertilised human egg. The combination of genetic material — half from the father and half from the mother — is then replicated to produce the myriad of cells needed for the tiny foetus to become a child. From one tiny cell comes a baby weighing several kilograms. Every cell in the body contains the same genetic information but by birth that information is expressed in countless different ways in their structure, function and location.

These extraordinary changes are determined by signals in the environment surrounding the cells. These signals come from a variety of sources: chemicals, hormones or contact with other cells. They spark a complex cascade of reactions within each individual cell that activate specific parts of the genetic information and deactivate others. At the same time each cell is driven to migrate and take on a specific task. By birth, the result is seen in the array of necessary organs and systems required for independent life.

Parents observe their baby's heartbeat and breathing at birth. The lungs and the heart are developed, fully functioning, and, like other organs, need only grow in pace with the body.

The brain is different

So if this new-born baby has already fully developed all these structures, what has been happening to the brain? The answer is unexpected. The brain, the most vital of all our organs, is quite

The World Begins

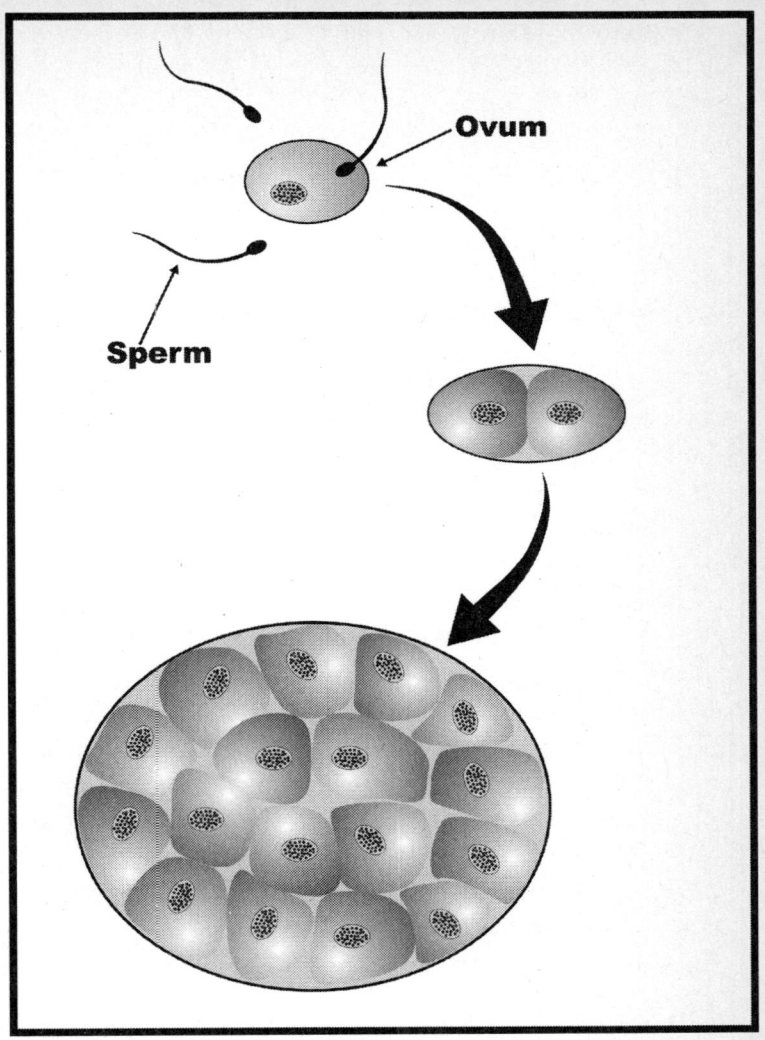

Fertilisation of an ovum and its division by four days.

different. It controls everything we do, think, and feel. It shapes our thoughts, hopes, dreams and imagination. To undertake the size of this extraordinary task, the brain has adopted its own unique solutions and develops with a capacity to adapt to change. Unlike other organs, the brain enters the world in a very unfinished state. The vast majority of its cells at birth are immature, not yet performing their assigned function and not connected to communicate with others. This leaves it flexible and open to alteration.

At the centre of these demands is the need to ensure survival. It is the one primary and over-riding duty of the brain. This reflexive reaction has fast-track connections to activate all vital functions required and to shut down others. Triggered by threat or danger, the heartbeat and breathing accelerate, blood glucose, adrenaline and cortisol levels increase and the autonomic nervous system is sparked. The brain is aroused and the body is ready for action. The powerhouse of this essential network lies in the most primitive area of the brain, the brain-stem. Necessary for life, it must be and is mature at birth. Its organisation is thought to be driven by the most dominant sensory experience of the foetus, the vibration and the sound of a steady maternal heartbeat.

While many of the mechanisms of human brain development remain secret, scientists have unravelled the enigma sufficiently to demonstrate a process that is stunning in both its complexity and precision.

The journey starts at just three to four weeks after conception. A thin layer of cells collects in the yellowish gelatine-like embryo — at this stage smaller than a grain of rice. This layer of cells then folds and crinkles like a piece of paper. Within a few days the crinkles thicken and fuse to form a fluid-filled tube. This tube forms the basis of the spinal cord and the brain.

The magic that drives this development lies in programmes encoded in genes. The process they direct is an intricate and beautiful choreography. If we imagine the noise a brain would make as it begins to evolve, then it would be like the buzzing and hum of excitement bees make around a hive in midsummer. This extraordinary racket shares the same dedicated sense of purpose. It is the crackling and the busyness of the bursts of electrical activity through which the forming brain cells begin to send messages to their companions.

Coming in co-ordinated pulsing waves, this activity sculpts the physical structure of the brain, laying down the first connections and, more importantly, provoking the brain cells to proliferate at the unbelievable rate of their maximum of 250,000 per minute. This feverish activity produces roughly twice as many brain cells as the brain will ever need. The excess is an ingenious solution to provide a safety margin to ensure that the brains of new-born babies are equipped with all the cells required to direct and contribute to their healthy development. Most of the lifetime's supply of brain cells begins to be produced within the first month of gestation and, complete by six months, those not required are shed before birth.

Another powerful control determines the ultimate function of some of the brain cells and directs the migration of others to their required locations. The process by which brain cells take on specific functions begins at approximately 14 weeks of gestation and continues throughout the first year of life. Of those that direct function, one encoded gene, for example, directs the cells that carry it to produce a substance that diffuses from the cells into their environment. Different concentrations of this chemical absorbed by nearby cells determine their destiny. For some, this is to be part of the network of brain cells that control the motor system of the child. Absorbed at a lower concentration it ensures that other brain cells become connecting cells relaying their messages to others.

In a similar way the genetic programmes that guide cells to their final location are being discovered. Starting at the same time as those directing function, a massive migration takes place when the foetus is 4½ months old, and tapers off by the eighth month. The cerebral cortex is the most dramatic example. The neurons already predetermined to be cortical slide up fibres produced by protecting cells in distinct populations. The last cells have to elbow their way through the established communities to form the outermost layer of the cortex. In providing these highways, each of the protective cells helps locate 1000 brain cells.

The power of the environment

The dance of nature and nurture is another part of this amazing composition. Although genes dominate brain development prior to birth, increasing evidence displays the effects of the environment. The movements of the foetus from a very early stage help to build the brain. Studies show that the foetus lays down memories of the rhythm of the surrounding language and of its mother's voice. Other sensory experiences bathe the foetus. Some of these are warmth, containment and physical support and the reflections of the routines of the mother's daily life. Another sensory experience of profound importance is the maternal heartbeat.

Adverse changes in the womb can also be powerful. They can derail this genetically driven assembly line. A graphic example is provided by the development of the cerebral cortex in early foetal life. The immature brain cells migrating to form the cortex must each reach their precise position at a specific time. Contact with other cells during this journey activates sets of genes, defining the eventual identity, function and site of each of these cortical cells. Any interruption can be devastating. Although most cells that go astray die, if any reach the wrong location and form the wrong connections, the results may be seen in eventual disorders such as severe infantile epilepsy, autism, some forms of intellectual delay and a vulnerability to develop schizophrenia.

The specific effects of toxic substances

Katy is three years old. She has been placed in day-care by a social worker. Her principal caregiver at the centre is worried about her constant runny nose, frequent coughing and wheezing. She is also worried by the fact that Katy barely speaks and does not play with other children. When they are excited, interacting and interjecting while a story is read, she does not seem to understand what is going on a lot of the time. Her mother, surrounded by other children, is always in a rush when she picks Katy up, and hasn't discussed Katy's problems with the centre.

Shane is four. He is often very tired at his pre-school centre, and displays similar verbal and social delays to Katy. He is also often out of touch with what is going on around him and has a poor memory. His mother seems caring although she herself appears slow in her movements and intellect.

Both children come from families with many disadvantages, and the major cause of these children's problems is evident when more is known about their homes. Katy's mother smokes and drinks heavily and did so during her pregnancy with Katy. Shane's parents allow their children to stay up until they put themselves to bed. They smoke marijuana every evening, frequently in the company of several friends who are often still present in the morning. They were smoking during all of Shane's mother's pregnancies. Nicotine and alcohol will have damaged Katy's forming brain; for Shane, cannabis. Each will be a continuing source of destruction.[1,2]

Persistent maternal trauma, poor nutrition, radiation, some viral infections like rubella, cocaine and other toxic substances are all influences that affect the sensitive developing brain. Scientists have uncovered the links between such toxic substances, their timing, and the outcomes seen in the children. Timing can be extraordinarily crucial. For example, a foetus exposed to radiation or cocaine on the fourteenth day after conception will have a worse outcome than if exposed the day before. This is well before many women know that they are pregnant. If these disasters are to be avoided, educational programmes on drugs and child development, including brain development, even in schools, are a necessity — not a luxury.

If the pregnant mother is subjected to verbal and physical violence, high levels of stress hormones will be released into the body, affecting the forming brain of the foetus. Such babies at birth are aroused, difficult to settle and over-react to any stimulus. This combined with alcohol consumption is especially damaging. Alcohol in pregnancy seems to alter brain development by directly affecting the forming brain cells and their input fibres. The disastrous results are increased by the unimpeded passage of the active ingredients from the mother's blood through the placenta into the foetal bloodstream. Once there, they cannot be broken down or excreted and are free to wreak their havoc.

Heavy drinking is known to produce Foetal Alcohol Syndrome, which is associated with a low birth weight, later growth problems, facial abnormalities and a range of neurological disorders. In preschool these children exhibit, on a continuum from mild to marked, intellectual delay and impaired perceptual, language and fine motor skills. Many have related behavioural problems. The advice is to abstain from alcohol as many more babies are born with a lower IQ without the damage being reflected in physical appearance. There is even growing evidence that alcohol consumption by the father can also cause problems for the foetal brain — possibly as a result of damage to the sperm. Ethanol also moves freely through breast milk to the baby.

Smoking can also lead to foetal damage. Nicotine crosses the placenta and has a direct impact on brain development in some cases by inhibiting brain cell growth and by interfering with the re-absorption of neurotransmitters, chemicals essential for neural function. Research has shown that it also affects the brain development of animals with likely implications for humans. That research showed that nicotine, at levels not usually considered toxic, altered the manufacture of the essential materials of the genes with clear long-term results. The links to the children exposed to nicotine prior to birth are seen in developmental delays, poor learning and behavioural problems. After birth nicotine is inhaled through smoke

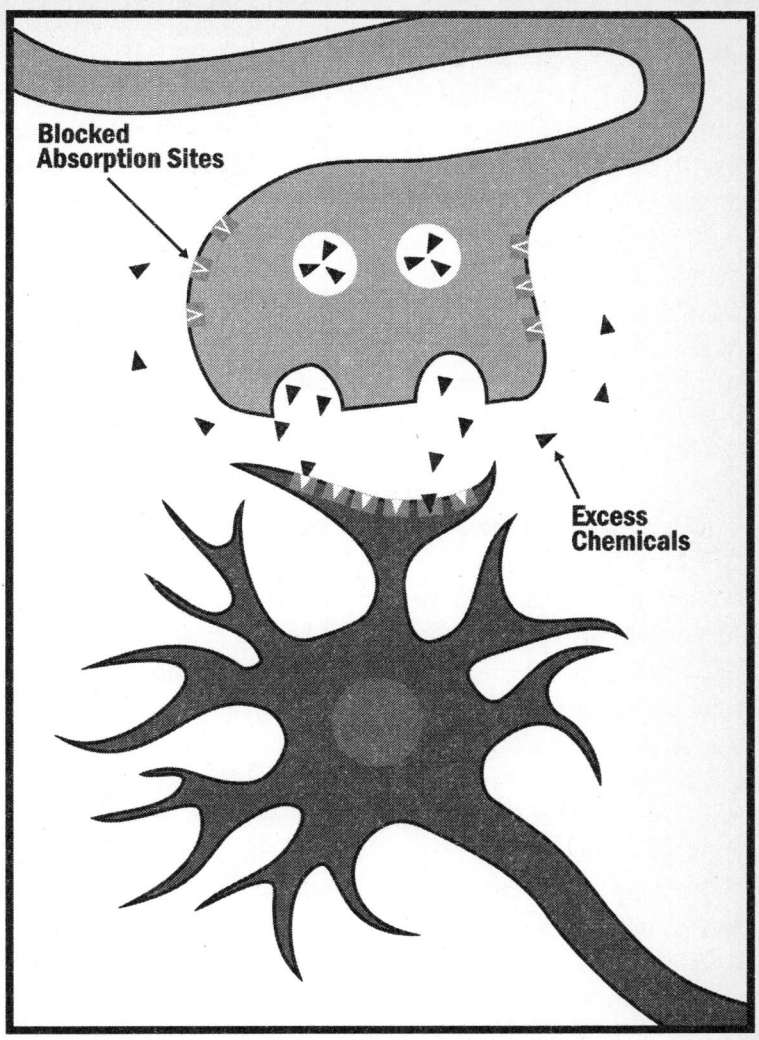

How some toxic substances can affect cell connections by blocking the re-absorption of neurotransmitters.

and enters breast milk, deepening the potential damage.

Exposure to cocaine *in utero* can devastate the developing brain. The primary actions of cocaine are as a stimulant mimicking the release of adrenaline in stress, and as a chemical with an ability to constrict blood vessels. In the brain it drains the stores of the essential neurotransmitters to produce the desired 'high'. In pregnancy it crosses the placental barrier and can restrict blood flow to the foetus causing a high incidence of miscarriage, premature birth and predisposition to cot death. The consequences for the foetus range from disrupting the migration of brain cells in the cortex, interfering with the production of connections, and inhibiting the re-absorption of neurotransmitters. Often compounded by other disadvantages, children display disturbances in processing information, attention, learning, memory and motor development. The poisoning can be continued after birth through passive smoke inhalation of cocaine in the form known as crack.

Research about the way marijuana affects the brain of the foetus and the new-born child has been added to extensive adult studies that have shown that this drug attaches to specific receptor sites in the brain. Professor Richard Faull and his team in New Zealand have shown that these sites are much higher in number at these ages and that they are located in areas associated with higher cognitive functions, movement control and motor and sensory functions.[3] Marijuana passes easily through the placenta into the foetal blood. Other studies of children born to mothers smoking cannabis in pregnancy show the disastrous results: they tend to be shorter, have smaller head circumferences, poor verbal skills, impaired memories and long-term behavioural effects. The effect marijuana has on cell division has been shown in one study to lead to a tenfold increase in later leukaemia. The fat solubility of the active ingredient of marijuana means that a single dose takes weeks to be eliminated from the brain. Smoke inhalation after birth and breast-feeding can maintain these terrible effects.

The World Begins

Fact file

- Brain development before birth is primarily driven by programmes encoded in genes although the experiences of the foetus assist in this development.

- This extraordinary process begins 3–4 weeks after conception with a series of events that lay down the first connections, but as their major action provoke the formation of all the brain cells needed for life.

Things to do

For parents

- During pregnancy a well-balanced diet, rest and skilled antenatal care help to ensure the healthy development of the baby.

- Avoid all toxic substances during pregnancy and after the birth of a child. Where an addiction is difficult to break, ask for specialised help. If possible, when a pregnancy is planned, embark on this prior to becoming pregnant.

- Ask for help if violence, physical and emotional abuse are part of your life. There is a wide range of possible people who can help your specific situation. General practitioners, lawyers, community agencies, family and friends are likely to assist or arrange for a suitable referral.

- Ensure that you know your immune status to those infections, such as rubella, that can affect a foetus. This screen is routinely given when booking for an antenatal programme.

For workers in parent education

- Expectant parents need to be informed about how they can protect the brain development of their baby and why this is imperative. Information about avoiding drugs, alcohol and smoking should be specific in its detail with assistance offered to those with any difficulty. Ensure that this is prominently displayed and that you reinforce this message in discussions with parents.

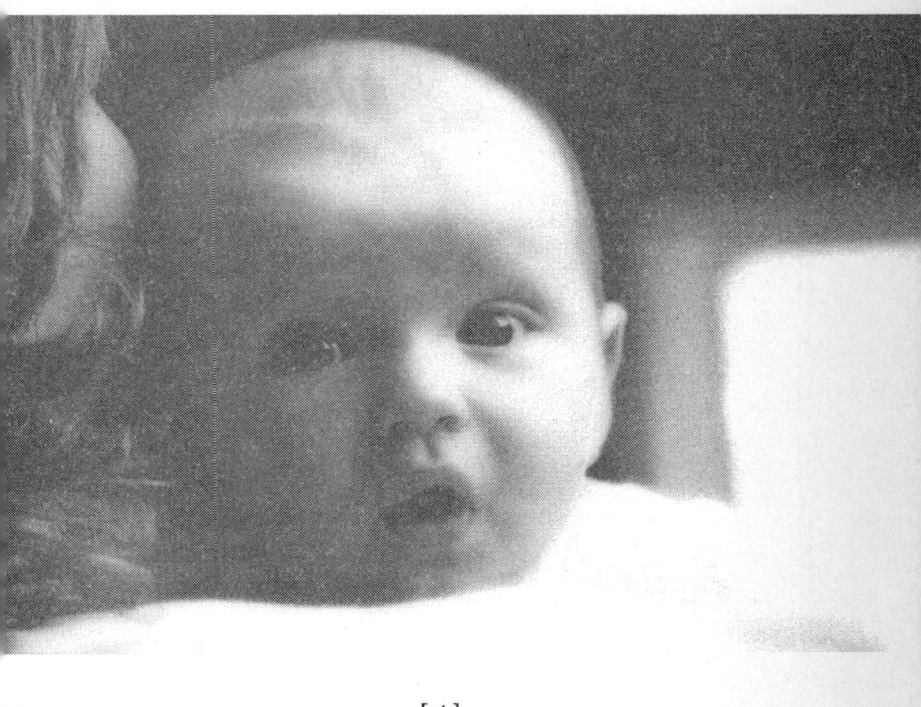

[4]

Potential and Experiences

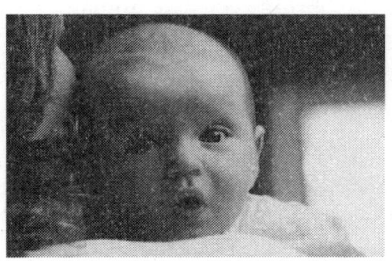

EVERY FIRST-born child brings a sense of overwhelming responsibility to their parents. The task is enormous and the questions asked about how best to respond to the baby's needs are as prolific as the answers. What happens in the baby's brain gives an insight into the requirements.

Before birth the forming brain's major achievement is the production of cells. After birth, development continues at the same staggering pace, but now in the area of developing the connections and pathways necessary for communication. Every ability, every skill and all capacities children acquire are developed and organised in the brain. Their physical foundation is seen in specific networks and intricate circuits of these pathways and connections built in defined areas. The controls spinning this complex wiring are the sensory experiences of children. The transformation of received experiences to these permanent highways seems unreal and fantastic. Understanding how this happens opens opportunities for enhancing the potential of all children and preventing harm to some.

At birth

Even the size of a new-born baby's brain is spectacular — two-thirds the size of an adult's. It also contains almost all the cells it will ever have. One hundred billion brain cells wrapped and embraced by 10 times as many cells that nurture and protect them like the bubble-wrapping of a parcel. The difference is that unlike other organs, the majority of these cells are immature.

It is this immaturity that highlights the importance of the environment in which young children live. The tasks ahead are the provoking of cell action but far more significant for the future of children, in the forming and securing of the detailed circuits and main trunk lines between them. The pivotal question lies in the command of this process.

The answer to this question is that the open, sensitive, organising brains of babies, infants and toddlers, are designed to adapt to their experiences regardless of their nature. This unique ability of the forming brain is highly successful in young children. It allows them in turn to adapt and respond appropriately to their very different and diverse home and family lives.

The day-to-day experiences of babies and toddlers are, therefore, critical. Children raised in a warm, nurturing and enriched environment will thrive, and, unseen, develop brains with lines for communication that will serve them well for the rest of their lives. These developed lines for communication not only bring benefits to their learning and behaviour, but also lower the risks of physical and mental disorders in later life.

The hidden changes

These daily experiences etch the patterns of the permanent pathways in the brain in a spectacular sequence. Like a spider's web, these networks extend throughout the brain linking the billions of brain cells together.

To do this each cell connects its long, tentacle-like 'output' fibre, the axon, to the projections of the cell next in line. These projections are designed to receive the electrically driven messages. Many of the axons have a layered insulating sheath, myelin, that speeds the transmission. This allows the messages to be passed rapidly and brain cells to fire their impulses hundreds of times a second.

The length of these axons varies from millimetres to metres, depending on their final destination. These heavy-duty cables are guided to their target cells by an ingenious method. Scientists have discovered the source in the tips of the growing axons which, like sonar guiding navigation under water, scan the environment for proteins that either repel or attract them. Sections of this special guidance system perform other tasks such as stopping axons from losing their course or from entering certain regions. This travel is often aided by another system that allows them to hitchhike rides with others. This ingenuity comes through sticky surface molecules, with additional signals helping in the decision of when to hop on and when to slide off. Driven in these ways, some axons undertake a journey the microscopic equivalent of kilometres. One example is seen in the axon of a motor neuron, which may travel from the spinal cord all the way to a muscle in the foot.

Pathways, circuits and networks of linked cells are formed in this way. Up to this point genes have controlled the unfolding of the brain, but once the first connections are made the sensory experiences of the child take over. In an astonishing display of seeming over-exuberance the brain forms quadrillions of connections. Like the earlier oversupply of brain cells prior to birth, the method in this madness is to insure that the brain can cope with its expected future demands. By the age of eight months, a baby has 500 trillion connections. By the age of two, a toddler has 1000 trillion. This is twice as many as her parents, with her brain twice as active. By the age of three her brain is 2½ times more active and remains at this level for the first 10 years of life. Small children absorb everything, process every experience avidly, with many, many measures showing that, beyond any other age, they are biologically primed for learning.

Compensation

There is yet another remarkable direction that comes from this wealth of connections and the ready response of the brain in early life to adapt. This is seen when an area of the brain is lost or destroyed but another region takes over at least part of its function. There are dramatic examples of children who are left without language after a stroke, but recover this capacity over time as the brain transfers this duty to the unaffected hemisphere. There have been children who lose an eye before the age of eight but compensate with better depth perception than those who lose an eye later. There are children who because of intractable epilepsy require surgery to remove an entire hemisphere and who grow the necessary pathways in the remaining side with the reappearance of their abilities to think and learn.

After age 10, the excess of connections is cut back with this diminishing the brain's ability to adapt to changes or compensate for loss. The vital areas of cognitive functioning, visual processing and the acquisition of language show that the first decade is critical in eliciting this response. If the brain is damaged after the age of 10, recovery is possible but it is slower, less complete and requires intensive intervention.

Practice and use dependency

Toni is 10 months old. He is proudly practising his new-found skill of crawling. At first he is tentative and frequently frustrated as he flops to his stomach. Gradually he becomes more confident and is able to move rapidly. He is delighted to explore — much to his mother's consternation who has to rearrange many precious or dangerous items. Practice has secured this wonderful skill. It has also secured, in a similar way, the lasting memory and the controlling networks of this ability in his brain.

The events that have gone on in Toni's brain come through a process directly reflecting his practice. This process defines how the experiences of early childhood control the creation of lines of communication in the mature brain. A repeated action received persistently over time secures a forming pathway. This stability is caused by the electrical impulse driven by these actions releasing a chemical signal at each connection passed. As the action is repeated each time, it increases the strength of the signal until it eventually reaches a threshold level. The connection then becomes exempt from elimination and retains this protected status into adult life. Conversely, connections and pathways are lost if the experiences that could have secured them are infrequent or neglected. This 'use dependency' is part of the normal development of the brain. The nature and the extent of the resulting pathways have a profound influence on how well children think and learn, not just as children, but as adults.

Pruning

In a natural progression the density of the connections remains high in the first decade of life with a gradual decline after this. By the age of 18, half of these connections are discarded, leaving the number at the 500 trillion seen in the eight-month-old toddler with this relatively constant for the rest of the life cycle. These connections and networks now form part of the permanent and highly efficient highways of the mature brain. This pruning process does not occur at the same rate in all parts of the brain. The brain-stem with its fundamental networks alters little. The cortex, on the other hand, must remain open throughout life to respond swiftly to situations

BRAINY BABIES

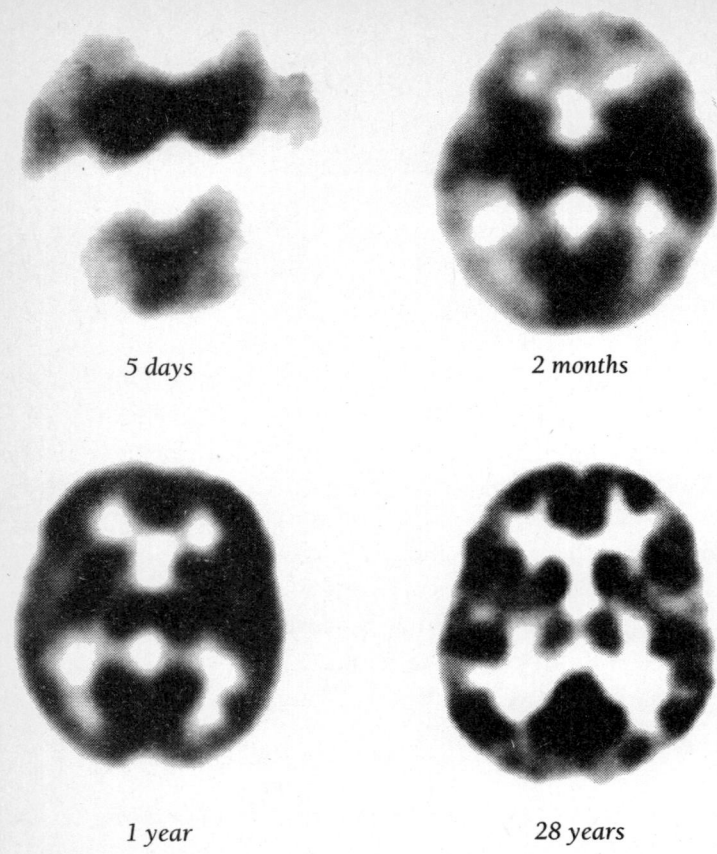

PET scans showing the rapid development of the brain. At one year it closely resembles that of an adult.
Source: H. T. Chugani.

that promote or inhibit learning. To do this, its connections and pathways are constantly made and lost. Any activity — talking to someone, reading or listening will cause this to happen.

By late adolescence the brain has declined in its ability to adapt but increased in its power to display a talent. A baby born with a potential for greatness encoded in his genes may turn out to have a gift for logic or a brilliant criminal mind, the direction defined by his early experiences.[1]

Significantly, connections can also be lost in early life while the brain is forming. The effects are devastating. The cause is disordered or neglected adult interactions. These interactions are those that deliver the essential developmental experiences. They are, at their best, the predictable and warm responses of a parent or a caregiver that are required to open the potential of young children and, in so doing, etch the permanent circuits in the brain. When these experiences are neglected or abusive, brain growth is either impaired or retarded. Very significant for the future of such children is the fact that this damage cannot be completely reconstructed or repaired later.

The power of early experiences

A mother reaches out to cuddle her new-born baby, securing her vision, reflecting a noise, a movement, an action ...

So what do we see and what lies hidden? For the most part these are the spontaneous actions of parents who delight in caring for their small children. A touch, a cuddle, an embrace. In this wonderful interactive dance of cues and responses, thousands of immature cells in the baby's brain are provoked to action, new connections are formed between them and existing connections are strengthened. The repeated, consistent, nurturing physical actions of the parent provide the sensory experiences for the baby. These experiences drive the repeated, consistent electrical activity of the brain cells needed to secure the pathways and the connections that will stay largely in place for the rest of life.

The experiences of these tiny children can add to their understanding and change their behaviour, as they can at any age. But unlike any other time of life they are additionally charged with permanently wiring the brain. Eventually this defines the powerful, secure and stable lines of communication of the mature brain and through this, influencing the boundaries of their capacities, competence and coping skills as adults.

By the age of three, the vast majority of the brain has been organised in this way. The first years of life are fundamental in laying a base for future thinking, learning and healthy social and physical development. By the same age, it is not surprising that children exposed to persistent traumatic experiences or neglect in early life carry marks in their brains that if not indelible are difficult to circumvent. Both the healthy and the harmed child demonstrate the vital influence of parental care and the context of the home environment in early childhood.

The sequence of brain development

The brain unfolds in an orderly sequence from the most basic area with the least cells, the brain-stem, to the most complex containing the greatest number of cells and connections in the cortex. In the same ascending order, various functions are developed from the most simple and reflexive in the brain-stem to the most complex in the cortex.

This sequence underlies the succession of the abilities young children acquire — from basic movements to thinking, planning and talking. Some are intertwined. One interesting example is seen in Sam, who at two was an active child constantly on the move, often demanding and difficult when he did not get his way. Now three, his mother is relieved that he has grown past most of this behaviour and is easier to handle. The hidden control of these prizes has come through the organisation of the networks in the limbic system and the front of Sam's cortex. They have a dual task — to attend to their own specific functions, and to regulate and modulate some of the unrestrained activity of the lower areas. This unregulated activity is expressed as impulsivity, easy arousal and a high level of activity. As Sam shows, this control comes into play to cause young children not only to lose this behaviour but also to be able to delay the instant gratification of their needs.

Some of this fascinating sequence in the organisation of the brain can be seen with one of the newer imaging techniques used as a diagnostic tool (see page 180). Positron Emission Tomography (PET) scans use trickery by supplying the brain with an isotope linked to glucose or oxygen, its main source of fuel. Lit up on a computer screen, bright colours in the brain show active areas and darker colours those that are quiescent. The colourful areas of activity are then related to the actions of the child. Repeated over time, these images demonstrate the growth of specific regions associated with different functions.

At one month there is intense activity in the areas of the cortex which control the motor and sensory skills the baby is acquiring. At two to three months activity rises sharply in those regions associated with vision and hearing. At eight months activity is predominant in the front of the cortex, that region in charge of the ability to express and control emotions as well as to think and plan. The baby at this time is making dramatic leaps in self-regulation and attachment. The transformation is extraordinary — from a newborn baby to a child of 12 months who is starting to walk, talk, reason and enjoy interacting with others.

The formation of one area influences the formation of the next in this process. Unfortunately, with stressed, abused and neglected young children, any poorly organised region causes additional problems later by interfering with the correct development of higher sections.

Other implications

Two-year-old Kelsi is causing her parents concern. They describe her as 'easily frustrated'. Her very effective solution is to express this in frequent temper tantrums. Two of the most recent ended in a loss of consciousness and a brief convulsion before she began breathing again. Frightened by this, her parents are now immediately attending to her desires and demands in an effort to stop these episodes happening.

Zak is four and has similar outbursts to Kelsi — although they are seemingly unprovoked and associated with defiant and difficult behaviours. His mother has tried many ways of controlling him and all have deepened, not improved, his behaviour.

The solution to rectifying such behaviour comes with knowing what is fuelling these responses and from which region of the brain the behaviour arises. Kelsi's parents need to be reassured that she will come to no harm. After a prolonged bout of crying, Kelsi fails to catch her breath and this leads to a temporary lack of oxygen to the brain. Without causing damage, this has precipitated her short fit and allowed her to recover. Her behaviour is part of the impulsive, demanding activities typical of her age. In the future her parents should distract her if possible and, if not, ignore her attention-seeking behaviours until they cease.

Zac is quite different although his outbursts are similar. He is a child whose behaviours tell of abuse and denigration. They result from the frequent firing of his survival or stress response. Sited in the brain-stem, these behaviours will not alter as this area is open to minimal change once mature. This automatic response has become the pattern of his brain development. As a result he is constantly looking for danger in all aspects of his life. His outbursts are caused by the sparking of the original memories of violence in his life, a process lost to any conscious recognition or control. He requires stability and support in his primary relationships and in both his home and pre-school environments if he is to have any chance to learn and to heal.

Potential and Experiences

Timing

Timing is also critical in this brain-growing process. Cerise is a baby whose interactions constantly delight her parents. At first only smiling, now she is actively soliciting their engagement by making sounds and intently focusing her vision to gain their attention. She has also begun to respond selectively to different cues and responses. Passing all the expected milestones for her age, Cerise is receiving the experiences required to organise specific areas of her brain at specific times.

Scientists are now able to define how this happens. These building opportunities are associated with specific periods when the brain cells are receptive to change and other specific times when circuits can be linked to perform complex tasks. These are time-limited opportunities when positive changes to the brain's final architecture are possible. These can be seen in different regions of the cortex which increase in size and continue to grow when exposed to the right sort of stimulation.

The final mastery of each sense and skill is linked to a set timetable. For example, those mastered by the end of the second year of life include binocular vision, emotional control, and social attachment. By the age of six, many of these critical periods in which senses or skill can be mastered are over or waning.

If timing is so important, what does this mean for babies born early? The tiny scrap of a body is engulfed in machinery and tubing and surrounded by noise and light. The tiny brain, torn from the security of the uterus, is assaulted by an alien world. These small babies are cut from the soothing touch of a caress and the sensory stimulation of feeding.

Not surprisingly, recent studies have shown that supportive care for pre-term infants can increase their physical and mental health and reduce the length of their hospital stays. While this is most effective with heavier babies, those with very low birth-weights and more medical complications can also improve with this individualised care.[2] Neonatal units are now faced with providing the special developmental needs of their charges, not just their medical requirements. These include less noise and light, intervention accommodating where possible the babies' sleep-wake cycles, reducing the pain and intrusion of some treatments, and a greater degree of physical contact and intimacy with parents. Cared for in this way, pre-term babies have shown improved patterns of brain functioning particularly in that area in the cortex which controls attention and planning, as well as more rapid weight gains.

Fact file

- After birth, the immature brain continues to develop in response both to genetic encoding and the experiences of environmental stimulii. New evidence shows how these experiences have a far more decisive and lasting role than was ever previously imagined.

- The pattern, nature and intensity of these experiences drive the electrical messages required by the brain cells to make and retain connections and pathways. In this way, they help define the architecture of the mature brain and influence the skills and capabilities of the adult.

- By the age of three the vast majority of the brain is developed and organised in this way.

- An early secure relationship with a committed parent directly affects the way a child's brain is wired. The consistent responses of the parent drive the repeated activity of the brain cells required to secure the stability of their connections.

- Babies and infants learn different skills at different ages. These are recorded in milestones. The information on brain development tells of how this happens.

- The activity of young children's brains is double that of adults.

Potential and Experiences

- The ability of experiences to control brain development brings the opportunity for insuring a good start for young children. It is also a challenge when these experiences are harmful and can disrupt brain development.

- The family well-being and how parents respond to their children are vitally important to their brain development.

- The early ability of the brain to change in relation to experience is also seen when the loss of a function through brain injury can eventually be assumed by another section of the brain before the child is 10 years old.

Things to do

For parents

- Talk and share normal activities with your child. Read to her as well as praising and encouraging her gains.

- Although children continue to develop skills at all ages, remember how important these seemingly ordinary interactions are in the first years of life. They set down the basis for learning and the successful patterns for other needs as the child grows.

- Follow the way your child's skills and interests develop. Attempting to impose different timetables never works.

- If you feel you have trouble in responding appropriately ask for help early. There is always something that can be done.

- Remember that there is hope for all children, even those raised without this foundation of a healthy organisation of their brains. Their needs should be recognised early and they should be given the nurture and experiences they require. This may be important when considering adopting or fostering a young child or when seeking advice for a child who could be maltreated.

For workers in adolescent services

- Adolescents, within the school curriculum or in community-based services, require information on the way the brain develops from conception through early childhood.

- They also require advice on the effects of toxic substances on the developing brain with an emphasis on cannabis, alcohol, nicotine and any other drugs they may be using.

For child health, early childhood education and parent education workers

- Understanding brain development is invaluable in understanding the requirements of babies, infants and toddlers. It also provides a useful framework to look for solutions when something is going wrong or when looking at the problems of children.

- Services and policies may need to be re-visited and redefined to follow these needs.

- Ensure that expectant parents and parents of children you work with fully understand the importance of parenting skills and the impact of those skills on their children's brain development. This must be delivered in ways tailored to their requirements.

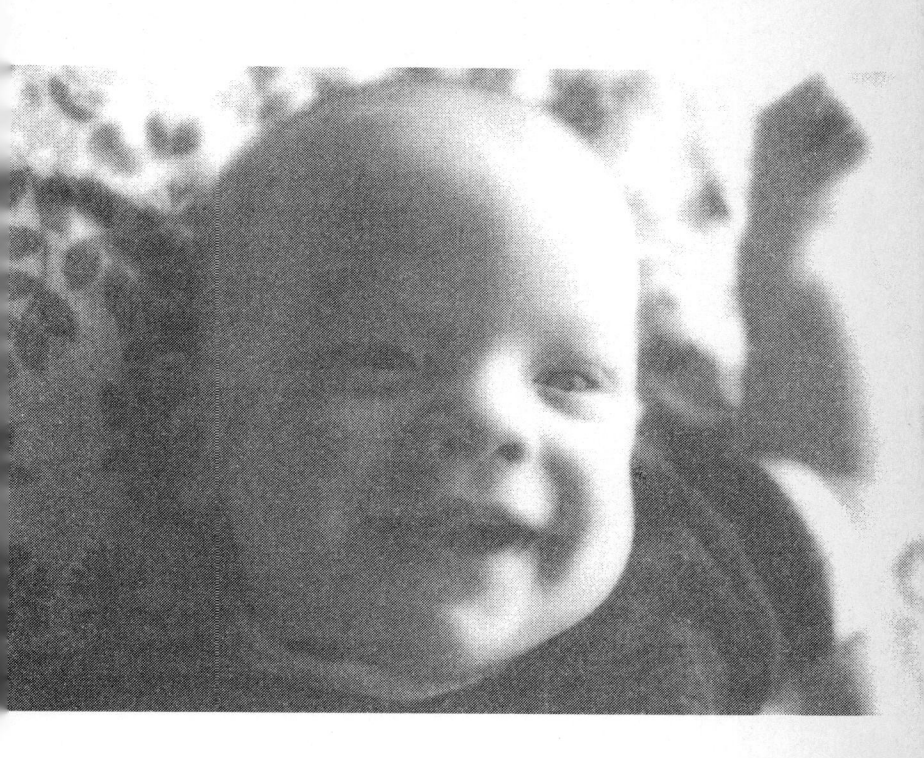

[5]

Movement and Music

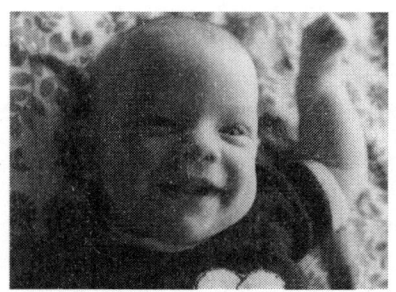

THERE IS a fascinating suggestion that a brain is only necessary if there is a need for movement — movement that allows a constant interaction with the environment in order to ensure survival. Chasing prey or avoiding predators are the most primitive of these needs. Translating this to the complex requirements of humans is the magic seen in the changes from the unco-ordinated movements of a baby to his sophisticated repertoire in a mere 12 months.

His first reactions — to turn his head in search of food when his cheek is stroked by his mother, to suck when he finds the nipple — are reactions built into his need for survival. These are reflexes that originate in the brain-stem; they are seen to gradually disappear as the cerebral cortex takes over to allow an increasingly spectacular display of motor skills to emerge.

Each baby and toddler is unique in this development as they are in mastering other abilities. Each young brain forms the connections and the networks at their own individual pace. The wide range of the observed milestones reflects these differences.

Movement before birth

Jade's mother is 15 weeks' pregnant. She and her husband do not as yet know Jade's gender but they are excited at detecting her first flickering movements. They are reassured by this confirmation of her presence and her life. Small bumps and kicks quickly grow to become visible and, as the pregnancy continues, some become uncomfortable for her mother. Her earlier rich and varied movements have been hidden. Beginning at just seven weeks of gestation, none are random but come in patterned forms with most continuing virtually unchanged after birth.[1]

Studied by ultrasound and video recordings, the variety of movements is amazing with startle responses, gross body movements, breathing movements, and isolated limb movements. All have been documented as to the time of their onset and any change they go through at a later date. The rhythmical breathing movements of a foetus appear paradoxical since at that stage the lungs are solid and non-compliant, the chest goes in and the abdomen expands. This pattern is seen in pre-term infants and can occur during sleep in babies born at term.

Sometimes motor activity is a response to the foetal environment and occurs, for example, when the foetus wants to change position. We see this when a foetus flexes its legs; when contact is made with the uterine wall and the foetus somersaults. This is an event never missed by a pregnant mother. The movement lingers into the first two months after birth when it is known as the 'stepping reflex'.

Other essential motor activity develops that is not usually thought of as happening prior to birth. Opening the mouth and yawning occur first, followed at 14 weeks by rhythmical sucking and swallowing. This drinking by the foetus regulates the amount of amniotic fluid in the womb although precisely how this is produced has yet to be discovered. Slow eye movements are seen at 16–18 weeks and are followed by rapid eye movements 2–4 weeks later and these continue throughout pregnancy.

There is accumulating evidence that all this activity occurring mainly in the first half of pregnancy has a significant role in insuring the proper development of the foetus, especially of the brain and the nervous system.

The working units — *muscles and reflexes*

Babies like Jade are equipped with the tiny muscles, ligaments and nerves required to move. Her motor skills have been developing prior to birth. She now has much to learn about regulating and controlling her actions and progressing from simple reflex commands to movements driven by her own volition.

Muscles, each made up of thousands of muscle fibres, are the working units of movement. These fibres are controlled individually by a cell in the brain or spinal cord, with just one of these cells controlling hundreds of fibres. They are the critical link — if they die or are damaged, movement becomes impossible or weak.

The simplest movements are reflexes — a fixed response to a particular stimulus. Their action takes place in the spinal cord. An example is the special sensors attuned to stretch found in most muscles.[2] When a muscle suddenly stretches (such as when a doctor taps a muscle tendon) these sensors send a barrage of electrical impulses to the spinal cord. These, in turn, activate the motor nerve cells in the cord and the nerves to cause the muscle to contract. At the same time messages are sent out to other muscles inhibiting them from reacting to the muscle that is being contracted.

At birth, Jade's movements were dominated by a set of primitive reflexes. As well as turning her head in search of food, her movements included automatic responses triggered when she was startled, grasping her hands and feet when her palm or sole was stimulated, and the stepping reflex. Within the first few months these diminish and disappear as Jade progresses and cortical function takes over. As an older child she will show other reflexes such as automatically withdrawing her foot from a sharp object while her other leg extends to maintain her balance. This occurs without thinking, just as her new-born responses were involuntary.

The tangled controls — the brain and the cord

Damion at four talks fluently, runs and turns without losing his balance, has learnt some basic swimming strokes and is very proud of a tune he has learnt to play on the piano. His movements are the combined result of many brain areas acting together like individual instruments in an orchestra. The type of movement, its sensitivity, and whether it requires conscious control determines whether the string or the brass sections of the orchestra play the dominant role. The dexterity of a master violinist or flautist seems a long way from the first efforts of a baby. But even a baby will quickly accomplish highly skilled movements, just as Damion has, as he learns to walk, speak and use his fingers precisely.

Once movement changes from the simplicity of muscles and reflexes it becomes more complex. This begins with the control of the sensors — those directed by their individual sets of nerve or brain cells that allow Damion to manage movements as varied as picking a petal from a flower to bluntly punching his brother. Beyond this another answer concerns how some muscles must be rhythmically co-ordinated when he walks or runs. As with reflexes, the signals come from the spinal cord.

The most complex movements, including those that are voluntary and require planning, largely involve the control of spinal mechanisms by the section of the cortex dedicated to movement. This motor cortex is at the top of the hierarchy of control. Some of these movements include those fine movements Damion acquired as an infant — accurately picking up a raisin with his thumb and index finger or learning to make sounds and then speak. Just as the sensations of touch and pain are allocated sections of the cortex based on the sensitivity of the area that records them, the precision and frequency of movements determines their importance within the cortex. As a result, the hands and the mouth are assigned seemingly enormous sections in the motor cortex while the back has a minuscule claim.

But not the monopoly

While the motor cortex is vital for controlling movement, it is ineffectual without the assistance of many other brain regions including the cerebellum, the brain-stem and the midbrain. The cerebellum is the vehicle with automatic gears. A loss of its function results in poor co-ordination and disorders of balance. It receives information directly from muscle sensors, from the inner ear signalling head position, as well as from the cerebral cortex. The sensory motor co-ordination it generates is the foundation of skilled movements that require no conscious thought. Learning to walk, speak or use a keyboard are all skills stored in the cerebellum where they can be called upon by the cortex.

The other specialised areas involved have wide connections with the sensory and motor areas of the cortex. They are a group of interconnected regions that exchange an incessant dialogue between themselves. If any of these regions is damaged, the consequences can be devastating — ranging from wild involuntary movements to a difficulty in activating movements.

The succession of motor skills

As the motor and the sensory systems of a baby's brain and spinal cord develop, she displays an elegant succession of movements. Tara, Damion's sister, is one such baby. At one to two months she begins to raise her head when lying on her stomach. Her vision in this position gives her the integrated ability to develop balance and hand-eye co-ordination. Over the next few months Tara learns to roll and, with increasing strength, to sit. This gives her some level of independence and the incentive to begin to explore. This is usually by crawling, although occasionally, like Tara, a child can proceed directly to walking. Tara is happy with sitting. Upright, she can see all she wants and sort out where to go. Tara quickly learns to pull herself along on her bottom. These skilled 'bottom shufflers' often run in families and, like Tara, they are late walkers. Tara's next success at 15 months is her first drunken steps. From there, it is but a few short months to when she is fully mobile. There are many different ways of acquiring these major motor abilities — Tara's way is no more or less appropriate than any other child's.

At the same time Tara develops other overlapping abilities. By five months she is able to reach, grasp a toy and move things from one hand to another. By 12 months she can bang things, throw and drop objects, and use her fingers adroitly. In the same way gross motor skills develop, Tara must practise and master the fine movements associated with the cognitive and sensory skills it takes to build blocks, sort objects and help herself to get dressed. Tara's capacity to control and use movement, like other small children, is amazing. Yet, as with all development, her acquisition of these motor skills depends on the sequencing and timing of various stages of her brain's development, beginning well before she was born.

Music, movement and creativity

Music is a delight to all ages. Young children seem to have a special affinity for it. Damion's home is constantly filled with music. His father plays the violin for a local orchestra and his mother plays the guitar and sings when there is the chance. When they play or a CD or the radio is switched on Damion dances, claps his hands and sings to the beat.

Movement and Music

Over centuries music has brought these gifts both in sound and movement. For small children like Damion, it can bring very special gains. Music helps in the development of their motor skills and co-ordination as they spontaneously dance to a rhythm. Enjoyed with other children and with adults, it helps children learn social skills and competence. Singing songs improves their linguistic skills. Enjoying the pleasure, they repeat their favourite dance or song, displaying their pride in doing something well with their parents' interest increasing their self-esteem.

The rewards go further as children discover and master their bodies through singing, movement and balance. It brings a sense of reward, and adds to their feelings of self-worth and confidence. As they mix these skills with their senses their creativity expands, spilling into their art, stories and play. Such creativity should be encouraged since it adds to their vision and capabilities as they grow, bringing the wonderful gift of thinking outside the limits of academic knowledge.

The natural harmonies of music have an importance in other directions. Recent studies with young children have shown how learning to play the piano affects the ability to link space and time, a concept that is later useful in learning maths, engineering and chess. Whether this is temporary or permanent has yet to be confirmed. Another aspect being explored is the value of traditional healing songs and dances in cultures throughout the world. Their building blocks, almost without exception, are the repetition of the rhythm of the maternal heartbeat that surrounds a baby before birth. This has led to a programme of music and movement aimed at economically disadvantaged pre-school children.[3] Children who went through the programme improved their fine and gross motor skills, self-help and expressive language. Other programmes incorporating music and other arts have demonstrated the same results — providing maltreated children with nurturing and enriching experiences shown to advance their sensory stimulation and their social, behavioural and emotional growth.[4]

Fact file

- The first movements of babies are automatic, with some assisting their survival. The range of sophisticated movements that infants and young children rapidly acquire comes through integration of the brain and the spinal cord, with the motor cortex at the top of the hierarchy of control.

- The speed at which specific motor skills are acquired as well as differences in the type of skills developed varies between children.

- Music enhances young children's motor co-ordination, balance, creativity and social learning.

- The rhythm of traditional cultural healing songs is the same rhythm as the steady maternal heartbeat heard before birth. These rhythms are being explored as potential aids in healing children damaged by abuse and other traumatic experiences.

Things to do
For parents and childcare and health workers

- Use music, dance and movements to help young children master motor skills and learn aspects of creativity and social behaviour as well as giving pleasure that is likely to be for life.

- Assist infants and toddlers in the movements they are acquiring by reflecting their actions, praising their efforts, giving opportunities for their use and talking to them about what they are doing.

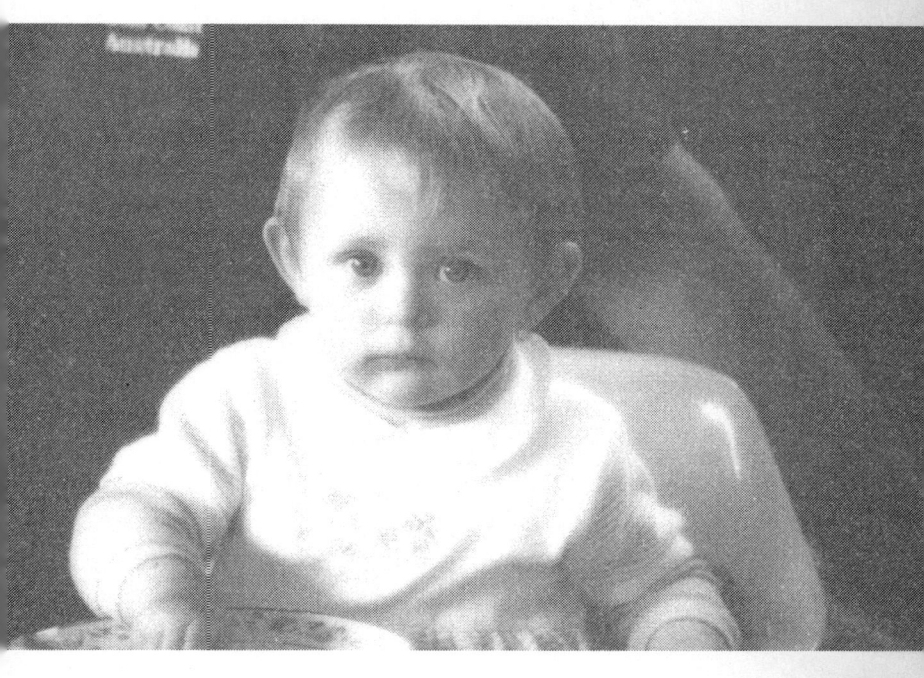

[6]

Mastering the Senses

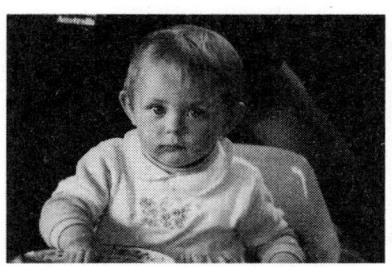

A BABY, new to the world, opens her eyes when suckling, to the delight of her mother. The eye colour as yet is indistinct as is her vision. She hears sounds as she has before birth and her brain is beginning to capture small clusters of information. Used to being surrounded by warmth and protection, she feels snug and secure in her tightly wrapped cover.

In a few weeks she will be watching her mother's face. By then, she will have amassed an extraordinary number of sounds, will know what to expect when she cries or smiles. She will understand that smiling brings its own rewards and will show her joy in response to caressing, cuddling, feeding and cleaning. A little more time and she will be actively soliciting adult attention by directly seeking attraction through noises and movements. The magnet is her irresistible eagerness and her directed vision. The weeks and months that follow continue these astronomical gains.

Prime times

Nicola's mother opens a book while holding Nicola in her arms. The book has bright pictures of household objects and comes with a simple story. Nicola is just six months old, but she is enjoying the sights and the words. As she reaches out in her attempt to turn the pages, she is understanding far more than she shows. The storytelling helps her notice colours, collect a memory of sounds and develop a joy of books even though none of these are yet an obvious part of her life.

Because the brain is capable of changing in response to experiences, different regions in Nicola's brain are developing. Timing is crucial in creating the circuits required. The primary areas open to change at her age are those of vision and hearing, the modulation of her emotions, making sounds and mastering the next stage in sitting and moving. The wiring of the pathways is best supported when the sensory input comes, as it does for Nicola, from several sources. This also helps strengthen other capacities she is developing such as cognition, attachment and balanced arousal responses. There is only a limited opportunity to create these circuits and once the individual times have passed for each of these acquisitions, the chances of forging these pathways are diminished.

For Nicola there is no concern. The way her mother responds to her ensures that she will acquire the skills she needs as each week passes. The mastery of these individual abilities and her senses are linked. As one skill is acquired it opens the opportunity for the development of another. As she is exposed to the sounds of words, she begins to understand them; her exposure to books brings the rewards she needs for learning in this and other ways.

This response of the brain to change and develop with experience has additional benefits for young children. Behavioural difficulties or developmental problems can be altered by appropriately timed assistance. This may be as simple as teaching a mother how to respond to the cues and signals of her baby, giving a child access to play with other children, or removing the source of stress from an overwhelmed parent.

From lullabies to language

By the twenty-fourth week of gestation Brooke has heard her mother's voice and will recognise it after she is born. As a new-born baby she is sung to, spoken to and rocked in time with the rhythm. Before she can mimic the movements of her mother's mouth in talking and singing, she is acquiring evidence about this in her brain. Before she has the skill to repeat some of these sounds, Brooke is gathering knowledge in her cortex of how to do this. Processed and stored as memories, they will provide her with all that she needs to move from making sounds to eventually speaking.

At first few of the brain cells in the area of Brooke's cortex which will eventually process sound have an assigned function, although some hold memories of sounds heard before birth. As a new-born baby, Brooke begins to hear the sounds of the language that surrounds her. This attention to sound is aided by her intense interest in the faces she quickly comes to know and their movements in speaking. Clusters of cells in her cortex are recruited to respond to phonemes, the small units of sound in a language that distinguish one word from another. Each cluster fires when that sound, that experience, is received. The stored experiences of these sounds lead to the acquisition of syllables and the rhythm of the language. Following the syllables, some words follow and are then linked to their meanings.

Brooke displays advantages lost to adults. For adults it can be difficult enough just to distinguish the subtle differences in small distinctive sounds that are unique to any language, let alone attempt to repeat them. Extraordinarily, Brooke at one month, like other babies of her age, can pick up these differences — and in many languages. If exposed to more than one language, she will only focus on those languages of the people she hears routinely at 6–10 months. Babies and infants like Brooke are not just hearing but listening. Parents help babies by adopting the melodious short sounds and a high-pitched speaking style known as 'parentese'. Babies' heart rates increase while they listen, and studies show that they connect a word to an object more rapidly than when spoken to in a normal manner.

Small throaty sounds turn to cooing, and by three months Brooke makes sounds — squeals, chuckles, gurgles — when hearing others speak. Babbling more continuously by the age of five months, she watches mouths intently as she tries to imitate inflections and learn how to make new sounds by changing the shape of her own mouth. By nine months she is responding to her name and other simple words and producing melodic double-syllable babble. Two months later she has added gestures to familiar words and has learnt their meaning by hearing them used in different situations.

By the age of 12 months the speech centres in Brooke's brain are ready to present one of the most magical of all moments: the first word, the herald of language. She has crossed the bridge from merely repeating the rhythmic inflections of sounds made by her parents to understanding the relationships of words to things in her environment. In so doing, Brooke has etched the circuits for hearing and speech. She is set to acquire an explosion of words and their meanings. Her specialised brain cells remain receptive and the next set of complex wiring is being spun. The transition from babble to language involves a bundle of emotions, reciprocated actions, and her need not just for contact but for active socialisation.

At 18 months her vocabulary will be increasing almost daily and she will be linking words. By the age of two years, she will be making short sentences. After that she will begin to master tense and numbers and, significantly, understand how some words can have different meanings depending on how they are put together with others.

This is the start of an extraordinary ability that allows Brooke to generate countless different sentences and use the correct grammar to describe her own experiences. Her parents will fuel these achievements by actively involving her in conversations. Nor does it matter if she is exposed to more than one language. Her brain will be able to easily accommodate and master different languages in a way that adults cannot.

Joseph is three years old. His parents are both employed by an international corporation involved in oil exploration. When the family shifts to a new country he is enrolled in a pre-school for multinational children of similar home backgrounds. Within a few months he has added the use of Spanish and French to his native English. He learns this far more rapidly than his older siblings do in school, and far more comprehensively than his parents ever will. Like Brooke, Joseph is at a time in his life when the brain cells processing language are open and ready to connect.

Experience will also build Joseph's vocabulary. A toddler's lexicon is directly correlated with how much he is talked to and how often he hears different words. Joseph's mother talks to him in all daily situations. She sits him in the trolley at the supermarket and involves him in an active conversation of what to buy and why. His father takes him for walks and asks him to describe what he sees, and reads to him at night. Meal times for the whole family are very social occasions. By the age of two, children like Joseph, who are surrounded by speech, have acquired a vocabulary twice as large as children raised with less exposure to language. The same is true for the complexity of their sentences.

Won't television do as part of this process? The answer is no. Children learn information when it comes with an emotional and personal context. The concept of 'more' will be learnt more readily when it is attached to the chance of receiving extra ice cream rather than being heard in isolation in front of a television. The content is also vital. Unlike television, parents talking to their child are talking about what is happening — what is actually real for the child.

Children not surrounded by speech are at a considerable disadvantage. Wiring the brain for language starts before birth and wanes by the age of four. If children's exposure to language is limited, they will not be able to acquire or practise linguistic skills. The effects can be serious. They will be cut off from effective communication, and this will interfere with learning normal social interaction and developing relationships with others. Verbal skills are also crucial for the development of reading and writing. As a result, any of the many language disorders bring high risks of other problems — academic, social and behavioural. If a child displays early linguistic difficulties, they should be referred for a hearing test and assessed by a speech therapist.

From seeing to vision

A foetus is light-sensitive from the sixteenth week. A baby born eight weeks early has the same capacity to see as if he were born at term. Yet at birth a baby sees without clear distinction, cannot focus and has no ability to judge depth. The magic that will allow him to look in awe at the wind creating swirling patterns in clouds or inspect the tiny marks on a beetle's back is one of the most delicate and complex of the senses. It also commands a quarter of the brain, more than any other.

The cornea and the iris focus the image on a sheet of receptors lining the back of the eye.[1] Each eye has 125 million receptors, each of which turns light into electrical signals that transmit the information about the seen image to the optic nerves in a very orderly process. The pathways cross before going through a specialised relay station to finally reach the area of the cortex assigned to vision. Columns of cells in the visual cortex react to specific signals such as perpendicular lines or edges that move. The final perception of such things as depth, perspective, the relative size and movement of objects, shading and gradations of texture all depend on contrasts in light intensity rather than colour. Countless images are disassembled into parts and stored in this way. There are no pictures stored in the brain. It is through these fragmented sections and the myriad of connections that the brain sets up the circuits to capture the various parts of an image when triggered, to reassemble these memories.

Nick is a typical baby. Very quickly he learns to focus on his mother's face as he feeds. In her arms, he is held at about 30 centimetres from her face, a position that allows him to do this. He can also track slow moving objects for a limited distance. This is all the vision he needs for the first few weeks. Progressing, he learns to co-ordinate both eyes. His brain stores the received images and weaves the circuits that join the movements together. These rapid gains allow the cortex to define the pathways and the connections needed for depth perception and binocular vision by the time he is four months old. Progressively these connections stabilise into lasting structures and by the time he is two his vision will be fully developed.

Because vision matures early, any potential problems must be given attention promptly. A frequent example is a child with a 'squint' — an inability to move both eyes together. Mastering this skill occurs in the first months of life, although some babies display a definite squint during this time. Questionable or definite, no squint should persist after the age of six months. If it is not corrected soon after this time, the brain will be unable to reconcile the two images and will instead choose to ignore that of the squinting eye, leaving a lasting impairment in visual perception. More rarely, children are sometimes born with a congenital cataract that develops into permanent blindness in the affected eye if the cataract is not removed promptly. The sensory stimulus of light hitting the retina is needed if the tentative connections to the visual centre in the cortex are to be secured. Asking early rather than worrying is the answer.

Taste and smell

Gary as a new-born baby has acquired some sense of smell and taste even before birth through swallowing amniotic fluid. By 15 weeks of gestation the taste buds are beginning to detect the taste of difference of chemicals in this fluid. At birth babies will selectively seek the smell of their own surrounding amniotic fluid. After birth, within seconds of Gary's first smelling his mother's body, permanent networks begin to form in his brain to ensure his ability to seek her continued contact.

If Gary is breast-fed, he will experience new tastes coming from his mother's diet. If he is bottle fed, the taste remains the same. The reflex that allows him to suck is present at birth. Necessary for survival, it originates in the brain-stem. By four months, Gary has learnt how to reach and grasp objects, to inspect them briefly and then explore them by putting them in his mouth. He drools as he feels the shapes and textures. He is also learning about tastes, about their association with foods and with anything else that comes his way. He approaches new tastes cautiously, gradually adding them to his repertoire of foods. This continues as solid food is added to the known taste of milk.

For Gary, as at any age, it is smell rather than the limited range of tastes detected by the tongue which is more important in these two closely bonded sensations. Yet, together they can distinguish thousands of different flavours. The loss of smell, the dominant partner, causes a significant reduction in taste. By contrast, the receptors in taste buds on the tongue can only distinguish four types of stimuli — sweet, sour, salty and bitter. When the chemicals in foods dissolve in saliva, they stimulate hairs projecting from these receptors, which then carry the signals along nerves to the taste centres in the brain.

More specialised smell receptors are grouped together in a small patch of the lining in the roof of the nose. Odours carried by airborne molecules dissolve in mucus and stimulate hair-like protrusions from the smell receptors. To do this the odours fit into receptor sites that react to specific smells such as garlic or cloves. These sensations are then passed to two brain areas, each controlling different needs. One gives rise to the smell perception, the other elicits associated emotional responses.

This combination of smell and taste can cause problems for parents. Ten-month-old Liz is unwell. She has a runny nose and a cough. To her parents' distress she is drinking but refusing to eat. Her temporary loss of smell means that she is no longer interested in her favourite foods. However, fluids are all she needs to recover. Trevor, a three-year-old boy with enlarged adenoids, persistently breathes through his mouth, not his nose, and snores at night. His mouth is consistently dry and his nose is blocked. As such, he is robbed of all but the most basic appreciation of taste and despite constant tempting remains uninterested in eating. With both Liz and Trevor, their refusal to eat results from the loss of smell not taste.

Touch

Human touch is magic. It can convey so many different feelings — from joy to commiseration, from warmth to disinterest, from cruelty to care, concern and reward. It is a form of contact that endures as a primary need throughout life but is never more critical than it is for new-born children. At four months, the foetus can feel touch everywhere except for his back and the top of his head, which takes another three weeks to develop. Their responses are seen in facial expressions and kicking.

With no experience of being separate from his mother, the new-born baby has no sense of any difference between himself and his mother who is perceived as being a part of himself. This central feeling is vitally important. A new-born baby denied the sensory feedback, and the continued reassurance of touch, can fail to thrive and will eventually die. Another rare but dramatic example of the importance of touch is seen in the unwitting but cruel consequences of infants raised in emotionally destitute institutions. Some of these children fail to develop any concept of the boundaries of their own bodies as they grow. They remain at the stage of a new-born baby with no sense of where their body begins and ends and no sense of their own physical being.

Positive, caring touch has other extraordinary effects. It is an essential ingredient for babies as an accompaniment to their feeding. As they suckle, they are caressed and cuddled and these wonderful feelings trigger the release of hormones such as insulin required for the calories from milk to be absorbed. Deprived of this touch, babies can fail to gain weight. Studies of pre-term infants in incubators, whose only sensation of touch was via tubes attached to machines, show just how important this is. Those infants whose parents were allowed to caress them grew more rapidly than those deprived of such experiences. In the animal world this neuro-endocrine effect has a dramatic ending. The runt of the litter is the one not licked or stroked as he struggles to attach himself to the mother's nipple. Neglected in this way, he dies, to the benefit of his siblings.

Massage is another example of the power of touch. It is a form of therapy used in many cultures and across centuries. For babies and infants, it can relieve stress, lower the associated cortisone secretion, and can calm related disorders such as colic, poor sleeping and irritability. Through massage a mother and her baby can relax together, enjoy the sensations of touching and experience some of the warm emotions associated with this sense.

Already wired at birth, touch receptors in the skin record the size, shape and texture of any object encountered. Where they are situated allows the brain to know where the touch is sited. Some receptors have their nerve cell endings free or in bulb-like structures; those associated, for example, with hairy skin are wrapped around the base of the hair shaft and are triggered when the hair moves. The sensitivity to touch and painful stimuli varies with the number and distribution of these receptors. The cornea of the eye is exquisitely sensitive to touch compared to the soles of the feet. The fingertips are more sensitive to touch compared to the back or the chest. Signals from these sensory receptors pass to the brain through nerves and the spinal cord to be distributed to the specific area of the cortex. Large areas of this region are assigned to those parts of the body such as the hands and lips, which are more sensitive.

Pain

Marion is a young mother on the postnatal ward. She has quickly learnt that the only way to settle her baby Adam is to comfort and cuddle him — something she enjoys as much as he does. As part of the standard hospital policy blood samples are taken from all the babies. Unfortunately, on this occasion the laboratory assistant was inexperienced and Adam was returned to Marion with bruises and multiple wounds on his heel. Adam was inconsolable and he took a long time to recover as Marion caressed and spoke to him. Marion knew that the blood test was essential but, nevertheless, she complained over the way it had happened. She was met with the simple explanation that babies feel little pain and the advice that she need not worry. Both the explanation and the advice were quite wrong.

New-born babies were once thought to have only a rudimentary experience of pain. This has been shown to be far from the truth. Studies have looked at, among other things, the internal responses triggered by simple medical procedures such as the heel pricking that Adam received. The reception and transmission of pain involves complex chemical and electrical processes. At the point of harm, special receptors respond to the stimuli of the damage. Chemicals released by injury to the tissues can act to enhance the sensitivity of the receptors and can result in more intensely felt pain. Pain messages are then transmitted with two different effects. Some are rapidly fired to the cortex, which translates these to a conscious experience. At the same time, other messages are suppressed by networks in the midbrain that, using chemicals similar to morphine, minimise the feelings and restrict their transmission to the higher centres of the brain. The benefit of research into these complicated systems is seen in better designed pain relief and medications, including those for small children.

Sexual feelings

As a baby Chas was held, rocked and caressed. He delighted in these pleasurable feelings and soon discovered he felt similar sensations when he held his penis. As he grew to be three, he often displayed and touched his penis at home. Curious about the same parts in others, his play would often involve him touching and examining the genitalia of his friend Bonnie, who was happy to do the same to him. Potty training was difficult as he was far more comfortable passing a bowel motion into his nappies, but over several months he learned with the help of his grandmother. He was never punished or made to feel bad about this area of his body. Observing his mother in the shower one day, he began asking questions about her body. His parents helped with this by reading him a simple picture book on bodies and how they worked.

Chas was lucky. It is rarely as simple as this. Most adults were raised to believe that touching the genitals was unacceptable; they felt ashamed of this part of their bodies and their natural curiosity was squashed. Spoken or unspoken, these are messages that parents unwittingly convey. It is important that parents acknowledge where these conflicts lie and look at ways to avoid them. It may be that you find it impossible to talk to your children about their sexual feelings. If so, don't do it. Instead, ask somebody who can. Share your problems by talking to other parents about their responses. Parents should never force themselves to comply when their own internal feelings prevent this.

Learning about feelings that in later life are associated with sex, begins at birth. During the pre-verbal stage infants have few inhibitions about exploring their sexuality and sensations. If you are confronted by your pre-school child engaging in sex play, it is important that you handle the situation calmly and avoid engendering guilt. Talk to your child if it is necessary in words relating to his developmental level, or wait until he asks questions before discussing such issues. Alternatively, an appropriate moment might arise, for example, when a pregnant friend visits. In this way parents can, from the beginning, foster for the children a healthy attitude to their sexuality, a comfortable body image, and open paths for continued communication.

Fact file

- A child's mastery of each of the senses occurs at a critical stage of their development and is linked to related experiences that the child must acquire and process. For the brain these are specific periods when the associated skills and knowledge must be laid down in the brain's networks.

- In a two-way process the child actively solicits these experiences and the adult responds, together creating the context in which wiring for these complex tasks can be laid down in the brain.

- The brain's ability to adapt to experience in early childhood also means we can intervene if for some reason the development of the senses is delayed.

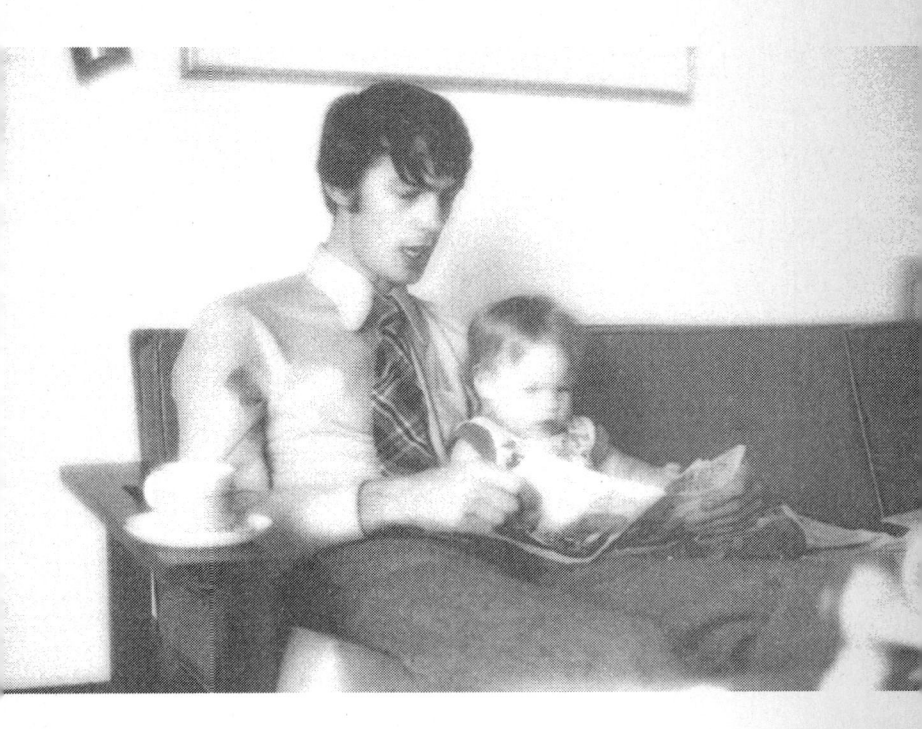

[7]

From Curiosity to Learning

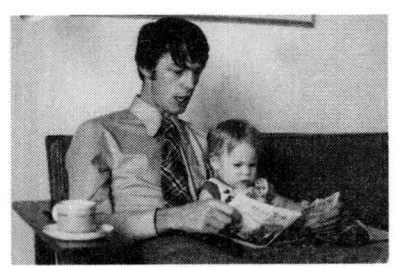

BABIES, INFANTS and toddlers have a natural curiosity — a curiosity that should guide parents when assisting their learning. If we pressure infants to gain age-advanced knowledge, we can limit the wide opportunities of their open minds and limit their childhood.

Small children are interested in everything. Tiny events not registered by an adult are amazing and unique. Water splashing from a tap, the purr of a cat, the smells and feel of 'helping' in the kitchen are all captured and processed. Their wonder at their world taken at their own pace expands their inquisitive minds and provides an extensive base for future learning. This pace is based on the stunning but immutable development of their brains. A parent's ability to share this wonder and the unique way children interpret the world is enjoyable in itself. For the children this curiosity wires in the associated skills, promotes their creativity and secures a joy in acquiring knowledge.

The social and emotional context

There is always something happening in baby Tia's family. Her older brother, Kingi, goes to school and the twins are attending preschool. Sometimes they bring their friends home. All the children are chatty, confident, and happy. Usually they are busy playing. Their play takes all forms: imitating, drawing, constructing huts, ball games, hide-and-seek, dressing up, and pretending. All their play is creative and will contribute to their wider learning. It is not that there are no upsets, fights, or tears but they are dealt with by their mother, Nancy, in ways that respect each child's different age and understanding.

These children are lucky. Their important relationships are providing the fabric for their learning. They have a secure foundation in their attachment to their parents and other caregivers outside the home. This has encouraged them to expand their interests and to develop an eagerness to advance on what they know. They are weaving lasting relationships and beginning to explore life, language and social learning, among a host of other experiences. They are, in their own individual ways, pushing open the boundaries of their minds.

Their play is essential and through it they explore their world. Repetitive games like hopscotch are identified with certain numerals and words. The textures of the physical world can be explored through the use of sand, paste, paint and water. Feelings can be explored and fears or concerns resolved through make-believe or dressing-up. Play invites thinking and reasoning as it throws up questions and discussions. As importantly, problem solving through play contributes to a wide range of cognitive functions.

As important as the home environment is to stimulate understanding, the opposite is also true when the experiences are negative. The enriched environments of Tia and her siblings are another source of stimulation for their development. Children deprived of this through poverty or parental neglect are disadvantaged.

Nevertheless, studies of children raised in poverty show that their intellect can be significantly expanded by exposing them early to things that are missing in their homes — toys, words, play with other children and nurturing touch among themselves. Re-testing the children when they are 12 has demonstrated that these gains are lasting. This is a powerful example of how sensitive the brain is to the environment and how early intervention can redress problems.

An inseparable part of learning is through the emotions attached to each sensory experience.[1] Children learn when an experience is rewarding or pleasurable, but not if fear is provoked. The consistent, responsive care of these children is seen in every capacity they acquire.

Learning begins for babies like Tia, when registered sensations give rise to an effect or emotion. Her responses are to this combination, not only to the physical but the emotional effects as well; a toy might be bright and interesting, or scary, a voice quiet and soothing, or frightening.

In the same way, adults bring an emotional meaning for children. Feeding may bring comfort and joy with a warm, attentive mother or fear and frustration with a mother who is distant and hurtful. These externally driven emotions influence children as they grow in all aspects of their learning. It allows them to cross-reference memories on the basis of the event and the attached emotions. It influences their behaviour in situations that come with similar emotional cues. The abilities to generalise and discriminate are learnt in this way. Long before a baby like Tia can communicate by speech, she will have developed a capacity to realise that a new adult in her life is frightening or friendly, and she will behave accordingly.

Play with all its disputes, rivalry and imagination demonstrates that learning is not just about intellectual development or facts and figures. It embraces social skills and the give-and-take of life with others. This simultaneous social and emotional growth adds to children's competence and the consolidation of other skills. Play can also be a critical step in understanding the way others think and react. It is the vibrant knowledge of living with siblings and parents which must be added to the growth of intellect. This is something we are increasingly overlooking in the modern world where technological skills are prized and humane values are neglected.

Flash cards, reading and computers

Sally and her husband, like many of their friends, are anxious to see their children succeed in life. They want them to be ahead in the competitive environment they will find themselves in as adults when they seek employment. Knowing the importance of early experiences, Sally has enrolled her two pre-schoolers, aged three and four, in daily lessons. They are now learning to read, studying maths and learning how to use a computer. Their baby sister of 14 months has flash cards and a special video programme using words and images that she watches from a sling seat. The video is one example of the dubious practices companies are developing to exploit the insecurity of parents and promote false messages about brain development.

The baby will most likely be confused when watching the video. Her brain will capture none of the messages in any useful way. Sally's older children may or may not absorb these skills prior to school but at what cost? Formal lessons disregard the way young children learn. Personal interests and enthusiasm are grounded in their own natural curiosity. Driving their inquisitive minds are the events and happenings of the everyday. Pursuing an enthusiasm in using play dough or the sandpit may lead to imitating their mother making biscuits or imitating how a building can be constructed. Adult interest in what children are creating can extend their experiences to helping with cooking or being taken to see a house being built from its framing to completion. Attempts to divert these journeys in formal ways can destroy these wonderful paths to learning.

Imposed lessons also disregard the unique pace each child has in acquiring knowledge and interests. Jack is fascinated by the colour of cups, books, crayons and the garden. Sally worries that this is delaying his progress but in reality he is absorbing an element that is important to him as an individual. Jack's later speech, paintings and story writing display this depth in his perception. Jack is also seen as a dreamer. In actual fact, he is not lost but is quietly focusing on interpreting the different reactions and emotions between members of his family. Jack's younger sister shows an all-absorbing delight in watching the habits of insects. This interest is likely to lead her to learn other vital lessons about different forms of life and the way they relate.

Formal regimens, such as the ones Sally and her husband have instituted, are likely to overlook the openness of young children's minds to their surroundings and the extraordinary activity of their brains. Young children have the capacity to absorb so much and to relate so much as they test and explore their experiences. This is basic to their learning. A broad canvas at an early age brings many later benefits when these wide experiences become the ever-expanding horizons of their understanding — or the limits. For example, by the age of four most children will have an understanding of numbers, a skill necessary for later competence in mathematics. Some pre-school children will want to go further and learn how to use them. Many will constantly ask the meaning of words and how to write and read them. Others may want to play a musical instrument. If the impetus for acquiring these skills is the child's own curiosity, then they will learn more readily with explanations, conversation, repetition and self-paced practice.

Computers are more of a dilemma. They will be essential in adult life but there are more appropriate times to learn how to use them. Although simple educational programmes are available, pre-school children lack quick hand-eye co-ordination and response to rapid images that computer skills involve. More importantly, computers deliver socially isolating artificial experiences. These are negative influences for children and should not be allowed to erode their involvement in the 'real' world. What is more important for children is their relationships and interactions with people. They are the grounds for expanding their opportunities in memories and learning.

Other avenues in early learning

Rua is constantly asking questions and seeking explanations from her mother. How does the vacuum cleaner work? Can she try to use it? Can she help with the cooking? Would grandma let her use the vacuum cleaner when she visits? Temporarily exhausting this approach, she moves to colouring in large patches on a piece of paper. Later she announces to her mother that it is a picture of the vacuum cleaner. Rua is using a variety of ways to express her joy in learning — her creativity, her conversations, her questions and the range of people and of ages in her life.

Parents and caregivers need to be aware of the rewards these spontaneous learning patterns bring to children. Some young children lack such encouragement to their creativity in their homes. Many children are excluded from creativity at school. Yet it is during pre-school and the first years at school that art and all its manifestations — drawings, story writing and story telling, poems and plays — are a part of children's rich experiences that not only enhance but are integral to their learning. The opportunities for the developing mind provided in exploring and expanding creative skills should be consistently valued and encouraged. Such creativity should be promoted at home — particularly if the school system does not include this. The benefits of a creative mind accrue not just to the child but to society at large.

Rua's constant conversations with her parents and others in her world are another source of learning to be valued and retained. The constant questions, answers and debate mirrors the classical and highly successful method of mentoring first advocated by Plato. Pre-school children, like Rua, rapidly increase their abilities to think and reason in this way. Their parents and caregivers are their guides and should continue to be so throughout their childhood and adolescent years. Our education system with emphasis on facts, figures and rote learning is not true learning but learning to play by the rules. This usually results in a lack of any long-term retention after the examination or the test has been passed. It is only when individual interest and emotions are sparked that a desire to understand opens new horizons. Teachers with vision can do this, so can parents. There are also exciting methods designed for preschool centres to do this. At school this requires the opportunity to test opinions and debate. Sadly, this is not often done except at some tertiary institutions, when the timing is usually too late for most children.

Rua is fortunate. She has frequent contact with her parents, siblings, family members, friends and caregivers. This exposure is typically severed as soon as children go to school where they are segregated according to age. Yet the fact remains that older children enjoy teaching their younger siblings — with evident rewards for both. Many older people — grandparents, neighbours, family friends — add so much value and offer so many different perspectives when they talk and interact with children. This has been the essence of child rearing for centuries. We need to redress this problem in our education system by encouraging such mentoring at school so that older children and other adults are encouraged to contribute within the school environment. In doing so, it would liberate another powerful source of effective early learning into the school years.

Reasoning and learning right from wrong

Bob was left as a boy without the challenges of debate and reasoning in his home. This has meant that as an adult he has difficulties making crucial decisions and planning in his business. He is desperate to see his young children learn the roots of clear and comprehensive thinking so that they can come to sound conclusions. Bob is well aware that what his children learn now will be the foundations by which they will resolve later issues they will begin to confront in adolescence. He has discussed the best way to do this with his wife Jackie.

Jackie's upbringing was different to Bob. Her parents would talk to her when she was young about a problem or an event in their lives and encourage her to look at all possible contributing factors and the possible consequences. She was also encouraged to listen to their experiences of others and the family would often discuss why another person may have thought or reacted differently to a shared or similar situation. Jackie also remembered how her father helped her solve problems through play, suggesting useful solutions when she reached an obstacle. In hindsight, she realised that she was often guided to the solution but left with the feeling that she had reached this herself. Bob and Jackie's children, now four and five, have already benefited from this approach and are now initiating play and many of these conversations themselves.

Matt and Elaine are appalled at the stories they had heard of two families they know whose teenage children have gone astray and have ruined their lives. They are keen that their son Matua is different. They know that the distinction of right from wrong is fundamental to his upbringing. In discussing this with a paediatrician who looks after Matua's asthma, they have learnt that the central needs are empathy, a sense of responsibility and moving the self-centred focus of early life to an understanding of others. Without realising it, they were already giving him this direction.

Matua at three loves his family. His sense of his own identity is now secure enough that he can understand what others may be feeling — the pre-requisite for empathy. This is reflected in the way he treats his friends, and with his actions endorsed by his parents, this is further strengthening his progress. Matua's early sense of responsibility came from looking after his toys and helping to look after himself. In this he was guided by his parents. The give-and-take of games and the controls placed on his demands has meant that he now realises the benefits of sharing and being concerned about others. As a toddler he was assertive and had a strong will, and although his parents encouraged the development of his personality, they also placed boundaries on unacceptable behaviour. In this, Matua was lucky. Another family may have treated his misbehaviour with anger or punishment. Instead, his parents' response to his transgressions has been supportive, seeking to modify his behaviour by explaining the consequences of his actions. This has meant that Matua has an idea of what is good and bad, what is right and wrong. Strengthened and challenged as he grows this will later emerge as a sense of morality and justice that will become evident in his adolescence and mature as an adult.

The imprint on the brain

The powerful effect that emotions and natural curiosity have on learning also have other implications for cognitive development. Rewards and pleasures stimulate associated circuits and wiring within the brain that extend beyond that of the information received in isolation. We have already seen this unlimited influence in the acquisition of language. The weaving of multiple networks in the brain is ensured by this repertoire of opportunities and this enthusiasm for learning. As a consequence cognitive, social, perceptual, sensory and motor circuits all advance rapidly and dramatically.

Endorsing emotions is the central theme in all of these acquisitions. Another example comes with small children learning the concept of causality, a key component of logic. A baby realises that if she smiles, her mother smiles back. The reciprocal actions produce responses that spark warm feelings for the baby, increasing her desire to indulge in this action repeatedly. Such warm feelings create and enhance the areas in her brain for smiling, for attachment and for building the basic knowledge of cause and effect. This becomes the foundation for more complex concepts of causality to develop over time. Amazingly, children as young as 7–12 months can link feelings and language with concepts based on this early blueprint. The same happens when the enthusiasm of a teacher for her subject infects her students.

Memory

Young children form crucial memories. They are memories that capture the events of each day in exquisite detail. They then weave them in patterns with other memories. This capacity to make internal representations of experiences is extraordinary. That the human brain can match and store endless volumes of these representations is even more remarkable. It is the depth and power of human memory that has allowed humans to dominate all other species.

Learning is, quite obviously, founded on memory. Our memories of similar events invite comparisons and solutions. When our memories are added to other memories, our understanding of things increases. Memories of the new and the unusual challenge the boundaries of past experience. Memories gathered from different perspectives can open hidden horizons. Some dart near the surface of the mind poised for frequent action. Others float deeper to be brought to view by an unexpected voice, a shared feeling or a passing smile. Deeper still are the memories of the forming self, many unavailable to conscious inspection, and others of trauma too painful or too dangerous to release, intricately and ingeniously concealed. So much of this elusive process remains unknown.

One powerful fact reinforces how positive emotions are central to learning. Vital for the storage of experiences in memories that can be retrieved is whether the consequences were reward or punishment. Our memories of fear and trauma are often fragmented. In their recall, they are not linked in ways that allow a clear narrative of what happened, and come instead with the impact of the intense feelings, the sensations and the physical responses of the original events.[2]

From Curiosity to Learning

The multiplicity of memory

Because memory is so powerful, some parents try to use it as a learning tool. How about playing tapes of foreign languages or music while the infant is sleeping? The answer is that these will never reach the cortex. Memory requires the sensory reception of an experience, its processing, storage and retrieval. This doesn't happen in sleep — it requires a conscious mind.

Every part of the brain forms and stores memories related to the function of the networks it contains. Those memories shaping the first months are usually implicit memories of abilities that require no conscious recall — memories of vision, movement, touch, taste, smell and sound. This is when babies and infants are learning to make sounds, to move, to identify the flavour of different foods, and look intently at a face. Another form of memory is called working memory, a form that is transient but allows retention of information long enough to reply. By contrast, memories of events and facts that are used in active learning, planning and thinking are explicit memories. They are consciously accessible records of previous experiences and can be recalled in a narrative form.

Scientists and clinicians have detailed some of the miracles in the formation and the storage of memories but there is much that remains to be explained. The brain seems to process and store different kinds of information separately. An area in the very front of the cortex is part of the system for working memories. Explicit memories use the middle part of the temporal lobe and another area called the thalamus. Other kinds depend on other areas — one, the limbic, dealing with the emotional aspects of memory and the other, the cerebellum, with motor learning where precise timing is involved.

The cortex is linked and cross-linked to each sense and emotion like a galaxy, a luminous band of stars that we are just beginning to explore. Still eluding discovery is the most fascinating question of all: how do the brain cells register these permanent changes as memories and form chains with a myriad of others in their recall? Various avenues are being investigated including the notion that with memory a permanent change occurs in the relationship between brain cells leading to a lasting increase in the strength of connections.

The amazing memories of babies and young children

Interest in the ability of children to remember has fuelled research and debate over the past century. It has been triggered by different aspects — from the lack of later access to early childhood memories, to the need to demonstrate accurate recall of events in situations such as giving evidence at court proceedings. Recent research is defining this extraordinary story.

How do the immature cells and the scant networks of a baby's brain begin to manage this advanced business of memory? The emerging evidence is startling: learning begins and memory is already functioning prior to birth.

As we know, new-born babies react specifically to their mother's voice and to noises they were deliberately exposed to in the last trimester. New-born babies identify with the smell of the fluid that surrounded them; they feel most secure when they are wrapped up and swaddled since this replicates how they felt in the uterine environment. Babies at birth have already developed a memory of touch and movement.

Research examining memory in the first six months of life continues this story of the precocity of early memory skills. Babies as young as two months can recall an event that occurred several weeks before if the memory is reactivated by some trigger associated with the event. They have a shorter retention than older children and their memories are also closely related to the situations in which they were acquired. As children grow these pre-verbal memories are signalled indirectly in their play, emotions, moods and their relationships with others.

This tapestry of memory acquisition is unceasing in its move to the more complex. Older children recall more detail of specific events while younger children focus on the routine and build this as the initial basis of their knowledge. Age and the length of retention are positively correlated. The context and the specificity of the cues promoting recall are other variables. Once again, talking with children is shown to be vital. Children's conversations with their parents about day-to-day activities and personal events increase the social function of memories and children's interest.

The loss of access to early memories

Why then do we later forget these early pre-linguistic memories? Theories abound ranging from those that suggest young children lack any personal memory to those that suggest we lack the ability to retrieve them. The sprinkling of memories most adults have tend to be limited to when they had learnt to speak clearly, although a specific cue, like a visit to the house in which their early years were spent, can raise some memories to the surface.

One partial reason for this barrier comes from the way the core of the forming self within young children is built of many memories that require no conscious recall. The earliest memories are those that serve the infant to operate within their world and to focus on day-to-day events. Any special experiences tend to be regarded in the same way as this base is developed.

Another possible reason is that this so-called 'infantile amnesia' has less to do with memory and more to do with the development of the sense of self. This suggests that our sense of personal identity only emerges at about the age of two when we are able to define experiences as personal and lay down these as memories. Another important recent study produced evidence that the maturation of specific areas in the cortex between the ages of one and four is required before any long-term memory can be formed.

The rewards

Young children are constantly learning — etching pathways in their brains, and creating the networks of associated skills. The experiences that fuel their memories are profoundly important. This applies to not just some of their experiences but all of them since the brain adapts to everything it receives. As children grow, nurture, care and warmth are inevitably mixed with disasters and daily stresses. Long-term protection, even in the face of major trauma, is founded on early memories of support, hope and memories directed to help children find their own solutions.

But memory has so many other sides. Memory captures the unique individuality of every child. Memory brings the very special interpretation of the world for every child. Memory creates the depth and the magnitude of such capacities as seeing, thinking and understanding. Memory is the essence of the mind.

Fact file

- Children's learning flourishes in the context of secure and positive relationships, through attached rewarding emotions and in an enriched environment.

- Play is essential to learning and can take many useful roles.

- Young children's own curiosity and creativity advance their learning, particularly when these are encouraged by their parents and teachers.

- Learning is not just about the intellectual acquisition of facts and figures but also includes a sense of self-achievement and of living with and co-operating with others.

- The brain moves from acquiring memories of routine events and those that lay down skills requiring no conscious recall in very early life, to increasingly complex memories that can be recalled and related later as children move through the pre-school years.

- Memory is not only the basis of learning but creates the unique individuality of every child.

Things to do

For parents

- There are many ways young children learn. These need to be understood and built into their home environment especially when they progress to school.

- Respond to young children in ways that respect their uniqueness as well as their age, temperament and level of understanding.

- Provide new experiences and bathe young children in language to enrich their learning, their memories and their developing minds.

- Encourage children's play as the source of their learning and the exploration of their experiences. Help them to do this both by themselves and with other children and in many ways — imitating, constructing, pretending and creating.

- Remember that children cannot and should not be totally guarded from expected daily stresses and problems as they grow. Help them learn through these experiences.

For workers in early childhood education

- General knowledge, languages, music, numbers and problem-solving should all be included as part of children's daily activities since they will more readily acquire these skills at this early age. Look at creative strategies to ensure this happens in your service.

- For the increasing number of children who cannot be cared for full time at home, good, affordable and accessible day-care is not a luxury but an essential brain food. Use the information on brain development to support this cause.

- Only use programmes that have proven to be successful to assist those parents who want to teach their children at home.

- Programmes providing disadvantaged parents with skills and their children high-quality early education have been very successful and should be set up in communities where this is a need.

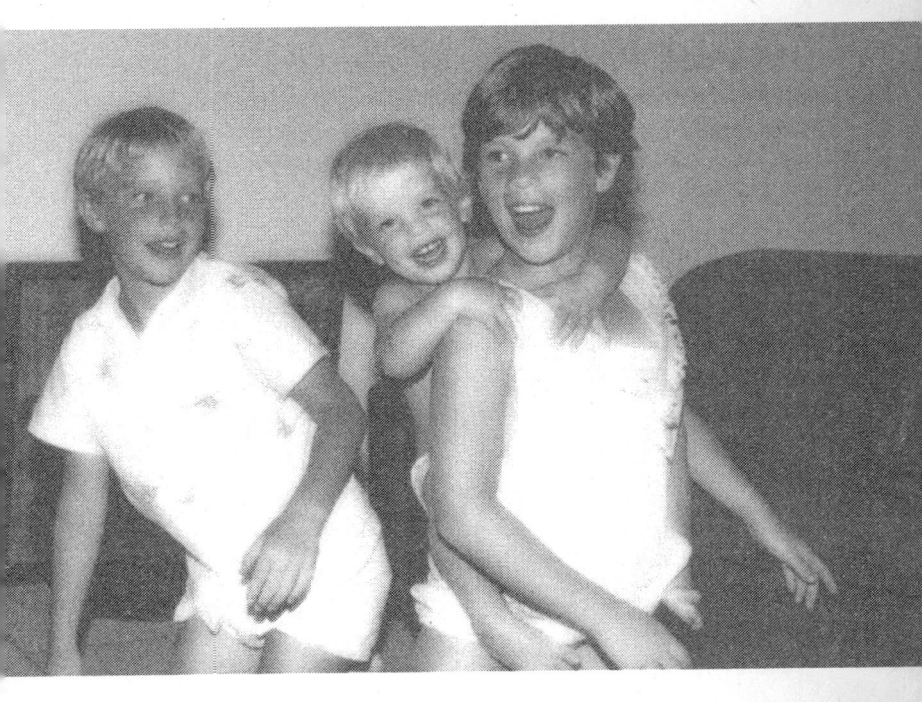

[8]

Behaviour, Boundaries and Discipline

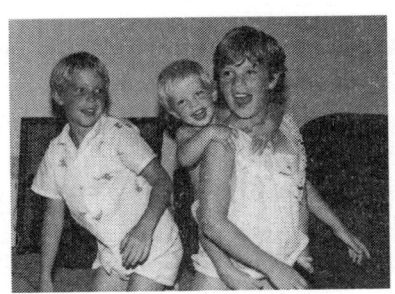

A T ONE week after birth a baby will show her contentment at being fed and her distress when crying brings no assistance. These emotions are among the first networks created in her brain. At just two months of age she will display more complex feelings of joy and sadness, assertiveness and anger. As her brain creates more circuits and new memories, her life will acquire greater structure and meaning.

As she grows she will require boundaries for her actions. Displaying behaviours in response to her feelings, she should be praised for those that are positive and distracted from those that will become destructive. All young children share this requirement. Firm, flexible discipline in a secure environment will inform her, advance her knowledge and help her to develop responsibility. In contrast, punishment can lead to fear and aggression.

Some of her behaviour will be fuelled by other experiences. Every child faces problems adjusting to their own emotions and to the inevitable difficulties and demands of daily life. Young children see some situations and events, inconsequential to an adult, as frightening. There are many reasons for this. It may come from a child's individual perception of an experience or because of the lack of knowledge that would allow the child to take in the true meaning. Frequently, it is the expression of the life-long response of the brain to treat anything new as dangerous.

Behaviours and discipline

Four-year-old Tom and his three-year-old sister Deborah accompany their mother to the doctor. In the reception area and consulting room they move from one activity to another. They show no respect for any of the books, magazines or furniture. Deborah pushes her way to the doctor's desk and attempts to climb onto his knee. Their mother disregards their actions and the destruction they are causing. The children don't defer to her. The unregulated behaviour of these children is worrying. They are impulsive, have no social skills, no sense of values, display a lack of security, and act like children much younger than themselves. Limits, explanations and distraction have not been part of their upbringing.

The repertoire of behaviour displayed by young children reflects what they are learning about their world, about themselves as individuals and their family. Initially, they are drawn by the need to explore their environment and test new-found skills. Gradually the skills are added to by others for communication and to advance their independence. Different children of different temperaments take these steps at differing times. These changing behaviours are the external expression of the internal progress in the organisation of their brains.

Showing disapproval, often not thought of as discipline, can be powerful. Rangi as a baby learnt through his parents' responses that he was valued and cherished. Long before he could speak he knew if his mother disapproved of anything simply by the way she would arc her eyebrow or frown at him. At three he chatters constantly. His mother shows her annoyance in the same potent way. If he makes a mess in the food cupboard, all she has to do is look at him 'that way' and he is anxious to make amends. It is the same with other adults who are emotionally important to him. The loving relationships Rangi formed in early infancy have provided the most basic motivation to respond to adult expectations.

It is essential that parents both protect and guide their children during these early years. A crawling toddler can find an electric socket, a cup of hot liquid or the powder for the dishwasher. Early curiosity and emerging abilities can enthusiastically spill over into pinching or biting another child as a way of expressing delight. Removing any dangers and keeping a watchful eye on these busy children are fundamental requirements. Showing disapproval and distraction are simple and highly effective methods of control and continue to be effective at a later age. A simple explanation can also be surprisingly helpful as even pre-verbal children can respond if they are treated with respect and understanding.

The behaviour we associate with two- and three-year-olds can be more demanding. This includes increasing independence, soliciting attention, sometimes in unreasonable ways, and showing frustration. It's this behaviour that Tom and Deborah are locked into. Partly, their behaviour is impulsive, aggressive, hyperactive and lacking sustained attention. These unregulated expressions are part of the unmonitored activity of the brain-stem and lower brain. It is only as the higher centres become developed that they take on an important role in regulating these lower brain functions in hand with parental guidance and the development of the networks for the control of their emotions.

It is important that parents and caregivers know that these changes underlie young children's behaviour. Temper tantrums, breath holding and other dramatic behaviour are normal ways in which some children of 18 months to three years or more express their anger and frustration. Giving in to these heated demands and appeasing the child only encourages more of the same. The child has learnt its power. Responding when the child is calm with simple explanations and alternatives are healthy solutions and allow children to learn.

When to intervene

Small children can easily hurt or upset others in their exuberant play. Tine loves day-care but today she is refusing to go. Her mother discovers the reason. She was frightened by the anger her teacher expressed when she accidentally kicked her friend. What she required was sympathetic questioning and an explanation of the need to apologise, however it happened. This is a response that will strengthen her evolving understanding of the need to consider the feelings of others. For some children hitting, pinching or punching may be seen by the child as a way to gain control, express anger, or to use its potential power. When this happens intervention is required together with separating from the other child and admonishing the behaviour, with reasons why the behaviour was inappropriate and other solutions given later when the child is calm. This can help children learn to respect others and to plan and seek their own answers when confronted with a problem.

At home Tine's self-will has led to struggles over eating and refusing to wear the clothes selected by her mother. There are also frequent squabbles between her and her younger brother. In these situations it is best to avoid intervening if possible. A child who refuses to sit with the family at dinner will not starve if other food is made available to be eaten informally. Over time Tine will want to share the conversation and the contact at the table. A child who insists on dressing herself in clothing seen by adults as inappropriate will not suffer. This is an integral part of individual expression for some young children.

The refusal to share, which usually occurs between the ages of two and three, is not worth waging war on unless necessary. All children come to terms with sharing in their own time. Teaching and reinforcing knowledge about caring for others should be the response if one child is hurt or upset. The struggle for assertiveness and control between siblings is a similar battle. For Tine and her brother, this two-way process is a vital element in their learning to live and co-operate together and later with other people. Parental supervision and separation of the children is only required if power is used by one child to harm or coerce another.

Positive and informing discipline

Roger is nearly four. Over the past few months he has become defiant, demanding and often impossible for his mother to control. Since noticing that he often breaks out into these irrational responses just before a meal or when he is very hungry, his mother has begun leaving food for him when he wakes and monitoring his need to eat. This has improved the situation but there are still times when Roger is difficult. However, she recently found that sending him to his room or even merely telling him he could be sent to his room, especially when he is busy playing with his friends, is an effective behaviour control.

Time out is a method of discipline that has its place for young children like Roger. Sending an aroused or angry child to their bedroom or sitting them in one place for a short time gives them the opportunity to settle down. Often merely threatening to do so produces the same result. Like all positive discipline, it must be accompanied with an explanation of why the behaviour was unacceptable and what the child should do if the same situation arises again. Such disciplining is only appropriate for children over the age of three — infants are too young to benefit as they have no concept of right and wrong.

It is no use disciplining a child several hours after something has happened. Children do not understand long-term causality. As such, if you are going to send a child to their room, do so for a short time. Similarly, simplify the number of available options. If helping make lunch is a favourite activity, then withdraw this privilege until the unwanted behaviour stops. Rewards for positive behaviour require the same attention to timing. Stars at the end of the day can be more effective than stars at the end of the week.

Roger's sister, Jo, often play-acts at being her mother with her friends. She not only uses some of her mother's words but her gestures and stance. This modelling of behaviour is often forgotten but extremely important. Young children readily disregard what adults say if they observe them doing otherwise. Ready to imitate, to learn, and to please – there is no better age than early childhood to begin teaching them in this manner. Jo has already learnt a great deal from her mother — how to help with cooking, how to feed the cat, and take care of her grandmother or their elderly neighbour when they visit. In so doing, Jo is also learning about the needs of others for comfort and care, in part by her mother's responses to her friends.

Corporal and verbal punishment

Punishment is not discipline. Hitting or spanking children is unacceptable. It may bring the intended compliance but this comes with the price of resentment, anger, fear and a reinforcement of the idea that all adults use power to gain control — a power they may replicate with their younger siblings and pets and are at risk of carrying into later life, repeating these actions on their own children. The less obvious messages can silently invade their brains to cause lasting harm. Some children become submissive and absorb their pain and fear. A proportion of these children, more commonly girls, become vulnerable to further damage, particularly if they are victimised in other ways. This can often happen at school when they are the target of a bully or a group of children who isolate them, or a teacher who constantly expresses disapproval.

Some become defiant, which if reinforced by other factors such as family violence can make them increasingly aggressive.

The persistent use of punishment also has other long-term consequences. Associated feelings of fear, pain and danger are incorporated into the social skills they are acquiring. In this way destructive experiences are linked to attachment and this colours any close relationships for the rest of their lives.

Our experiences as children can sometimes become the templates of our behaviour as adults. This is apparent, for example, in the way the reflexive actions of adults when aroused come automatically from the way they were treated as children. A father arrives home after a bad day at work to the sound of his children playing loud music. His immediate reaction is to shout at the children, hit them and demand that they go to their rooms — the response he had in his childhood.

This father shouted at his children. Shouting and denigration are just as punitive as hitting. These injuries are unseen but long term are just as dangerous. Children repeatedly told they are useless, dumb and ugly learn to believe this. Children constantly shouted at feel powerless or adopt this behaviour themselves in response to situations they want to control. As adults they begin to do the same to their children — and so a vicious, silent cycle of punishment, fear and humiliation is perpetuated. It is a pervasive form of emotional and psychological damage. We see it in the supermarket when a mother openly berates her child or when a neighbour shouts at her children with cruel and wounding words. Yet how often is there a response on behalf of the children?

Punishment of any form that is persistently used to hurt children brings risks of lasting disadvantages and disabilities. The scars are burnt into the brain-stem. The persistent firing of the survival response of 'freeze, flight or fight', driven by the consistent fear and terror, ensures that this becomes the pattern for brain development for both young and older children. It is a pattern that will alter their perception of all other experiences — a perception that tells of danger and of harm in every aspect of their lives. The consequences are many and all are damaging.

Boundaries and limits

Just as young children require information and direction from their parents, they also require boundaries. These are the known limits of behaviour, of territory, of articles available for play and exploration, of relationships with their siblings and friends as well as a clear demarcation between adults and children in the family. These boundaries change to meet the inevitable changes in children's needs as they grow and they become a part of the organisation of children's lives. Accompanied by care and nurture, they help to control children's focus on self-gain and anger while assisting the brain in building in the control and regulation of these primary emotions. As part of the organisation of children's lives, they teach children responsibility and respect, and assist in the growth of self-confidence.

The failure to impose any limits can be displayed in many ways. In a household where there are no real boundaries between adults and children, children can have unreasonable demands placed on them — demands that are beyond their developmental age and that rob them of their childhood. In families where parents fail to deliver any direction, unregulated early behaviour can persist, eroding the children's chances of social and educational learning. Just as deprivation can stunt development, over-stimulation can cause a child to become confused, anxious, unable to cope or concentrate, and have a low self-esteem. Children indulged with material possessions, but without any nurture and compassion, are at risk of becoming adults who have no empathy with others, and whose only interest is money and the external display of wealth.

In the first few months after birth parents filter the sensory experiences of their babies, defining the boundaries between stimulation and the need for rest. As the child grows other family members and caregivers continue to deliver these changing limits. Young children differ in their need for boundaries. Some are easily over-stimulated while others are less reactive. Those who require strict limits also need extra warmth and compassion. The structure and the limits built into the everyday experiences of infants and toddlers in gentle but consistent ways will allow them, as they become verbal, to impose their own boundaries. Some older children, for example, encouraged by their parents in discussion, will determine for themselves what form of discipline is appropriate for a particular misbehaviour, and are more likely to comply when this happens.

Fact file

- The emotions expressed by babies and infants are laid down in the neural networks in each section of their developing brains and are part of their memories of the related experiences.

- The behaviours young children display move from acquiring the basic life skills to the need for exploring and responding to their own desires and demands. Regulated in firm but gentle ways and accompanied by warmth and security, boundaries help them develop a control of their responses and emotions.

- Children need limits and if they are unregulated they will not progress. Many children find the lack of boundaries frightening — it can make them insecure and damage their relationship with others.

Things to do

For parents

- Children model and imitate adult behaviours. Parents and caregivers need to remember this and use it when possible to assist young children's learning.

- Punishment, which harms children physically or verbally, is unacceptable. If persistent, both forms can cause long-term damage to the brain, reflected in the way children see their world and respond in other social settings.

- Time out, the withdrawal of privileges for misbehaviour, and the bestowal of privileges for good behaviour are useful techniques for some three- to five-year-olds.

For health, early education and childcare workers

- Ensure that your service has defined pathways for recognising young children who are being harmed by punishment and for any other cause or disability that undermines their learning.

- Avoid directly confronting parents who persistently punish their children. Instead, suggest that the child should be referred to a specialist for some other difficulty — this may open the door to providing the assistance the family requires.

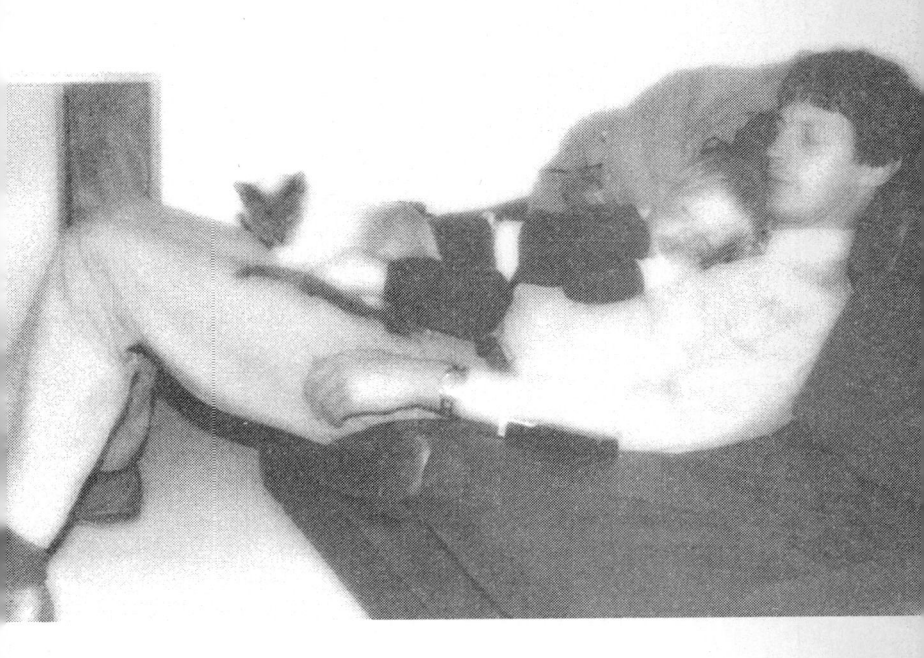

[9]

Sleeping and Dreaming

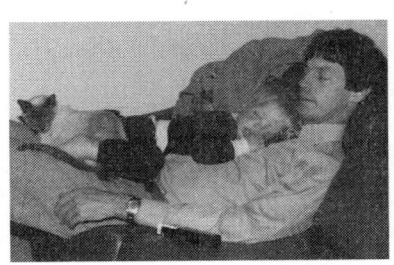

IS CONSCIOUSNESS the heart of the human mind? It has yet to be clearly defined by philosophers or scientists. Is sleep the restoration of the human mind? Some of its mysteries have been exposed but many swirl without capture. The feelings of calm as worries are left behind, the lapse into timelessness, the abandonment of any self-awareness or control? For babies, what are the feelings and the magic? What do babies experience when they sleep?

The basis of scientific knowledge

A third of a lifetime is spent in sleep. What happens in these hours was first explored in adults by recording brain waves and muscle tone. A major breakthrough came when scientists discovered rapid eye movement (REM) sleep, an active period characterised by intense brain activity and bursts of eye movements.[1] This is the time of dreaming, with the brain alert and creating its own inner world while at the same time the body is paralysed. The messages that create REM sleep are sent from an area in the brain-stem to the cortex to stimulate dreaming and, simultaneously, to the spinal cord to inhibit movement. This active sleep seems to be very important. Studies have shown that deliberately waking adults in this state is followed by desperate attempts to compensate.

The second type of sleep — non-REM — is quieter with a fall in the blood pressure, heart rate and metabolism, and comes in four progressively deeper stages. These two types of sleep, the active and the quiet, alternate throughout the night.

The functions of sleep are another question. There must be some enormous benefits to losing the conscious mind in this way for so much of each day. One recent discovery is that this is the time when the brain cells make proteins in a greater quantity than when awake. These proteins are essential to maintain their function. Another recent discovery is that during sleep the brain manufactures and stockpiles neurotransmitters, the chemical systems essential to the passage of the brain cell messages to be used the next day.

The onset of sleep

Eru and his wife are at the end of their tether in trying to get their one-year-old son Conrad to sleep. He refuses to lie down without first being cuddled and then having one of them lie beside him. Even then they have to wait a long time before they can leave his room and all too often he wakes up when they go. They have found that a drive in the car will cause him to sleep but he often wakes up when they shift him from the car to his bed. Advice from others has not helped. What makes it so frustrating is that he was a good sleeper until two months ago when he developed an ear infection.

Precisely how sleep occurs remains uncertain. Two mechanisms appear to have some role in the regulation between sleep and wakefulness. The first is in a biological clock — a group of brain cells the size of a pinhead in the hypothalamus. It determines wake-up times in a highly predictable manner but has more indirect bearing on when we fall asleep. The cue to activate waking is the amount of light entering the eye. It promotes wakefulness for roughly half of the day in older children and adults. The second mechanism comes through the body's natural tendency to seek a balance — this results in us feeling sleepy after a period of extended wakefulness. Research is underway into the chemicals and connections involved in wakefulness or sleep.

None of this will help Conrad's parents. His previous routine of a story, a cuddle, and quiet music in his room has been broken. He now expects other attention — being lifted, cuddled, fed and talked to. Leading him back to his past sleeping pattern will come with the gradual withdrawal of these extra privileges and by reassuring him when he wakes — something that will also gradually be withdrawn over time. This reassurance will depend on Conrad's responses and the choice of his parents. It may be rubbing his back or talking to him quietly. Feeding should be avoided as this can be very disruptive. The child wakes to drink and often later again to pass a bowel motion. Leaving him to cry until he is exhausted and falls asleep, although recommended by some, is difficult for parents to tolerate and can make a child distressed and alarmed.

The patterns of sleep

Replete and content, David, like other babies, fell asleep after feeding. David's parents noticed that as a baby he displayed differences in his movements, sounds and breathing in sleep. Unknown to them was the hidden maturation and control of his brain. At the age of three months David showed a more predictable pattern in his sleeping and waking. At six months he even stopped taking the one night feed he had previously demanded. To their relief, their interrupted nights had ended although other routines associated with sleep were needed, such as a story and a cuddle.

The sleep patterns of the foetus, babies, infants and toddlers are quite different. Rhythmical periods of activity and quiescence have been identified at 28–32 weeks of gestation. Pre-term babies born at these ages show active (REM) sleep with its associated eye movements and irregular respiration. This active sleep is dominant with quiet (non-REM) sleep increasing in length until it overtakes active sleep at about three months. At the same time sleep behaviour takes on a more mature form. As the neural networks mature, active and quiet sleep alternate more consistently and a regular daily cycle is established. David's development followed this pattern. His daytime sleep soon became well-defined naps and he became a heavy sleeper, rarely waking. This is often first found in babies between two and nine months, with 'good' sleepers infrequently waking, whereas poor sleepers do.

David's parents were initially worried about his irregular breathing and whether this was a precursor of possible cot death. Reassured by their doctor, they read more information on the way babies sleep. What they found was that, unlike adults, babies like David enter sleep in the active phase. They then watched this fascinating progress. David would fall asleep after feeding, his eyes at first open, his face relaxed, with a few movements of his arms or legs. His parents noticed that he went to sleep more rapidly when lying on his stomach. Despite this, they persisted in getting him to sleep on his back, knowing this would decrease any risk of cot death.

In this sleeping state he made sucking noises, his breathing became irregular and eye movements could be seen under his eyelids. On occasions he would make short sounds, move his fingers and infrequently have large, short jerks of his body. Once when his mother picked him up when he was like this, he was floppy with no muscle tone and quickly awoke. Normally, after about half an hour, his respiration became regular, his eye movements stopped, and he made very few slow movements. He occasionally took a large sighing breath and then stopped breathing for 5–10 seconds before recommencing regular breathing. Any noise caused him to startle but if moved he remained asleep. These cycles of changes continued, the active sleep more dominant, until he awoke crying and hungry.

By the age of one David was ready to be taught to initiate sleep on his own after a chosen routine with one of his parents reading to him or hugging him. Like other children treated in this way, he developed a good sleeping pattern as a toddler. He often woke several times at night, as do adults, but he usually went back to sleep unheeded. David's parents knew that there would be gradual changes after this. The overall pattern from the ages of two to five is that of a shorter sleep time with less active sleep as the child grows, and no daytime sleeping. Although varying between individuals, the optimal sleep times at various ages have been defined as 16–18 hours a day for a new-born baby, 12–14 hours for an infant of one, and 9–10 hours for a 12 year-old. Adults need less, with the hours often decreasing as they age.

Dreams

Although sleep is often thought to be a time of rest and passive retreat, it is in fact the opposite. During active sleep we dream. The brain is hyper-alert, the senses are evoking a flurry of sights and sounds, the muscles tensing and relaxing, while blood pressure and temperature rises and falls. Even so, we are not sure why we dream. Does it allow a journey into the deepest thoughts and emotions? Is it a chance to review the events of the day with others already stored in memory? We don't even know if babies dream. But why not? They have an enormous number of gathered experiences to sort, mingle and compare.

Fact file

- The sleeping stages of both active and quiet sleep begin before birth.

- Babies do not have a regular sleep/wake pattern until they are approximately 12 weeks old when the brain systems involved are mature.

- A child who is unwell will have their normal sleep pattern disrupted. Any attempts to re-establish their sleeping pattern will need to wait until they are better.

- We do not know whether dreaming occurs in babies and infants but it is highly likely to be a part of their active sleep as it is in older children and adults.

Things to do

For parents and childcare workers

- During the first three months of a baby's life, anticipate periods of wakefulness at night and early morning waking, especially for feeding and changing. Ensure that your responses are consistent and appropriate — this will help the baby change his sleeping pattern.

- Having rituals at bedtime can be comforting for young children. These can include reading or talking with a parent prior to settling down at a regular time.

- Reconstructing a disrupted sleep pattern after an illness requires a shared plan by parents. Re-establish old habits by gradually withdrawing the extra attention the child has come to expect.

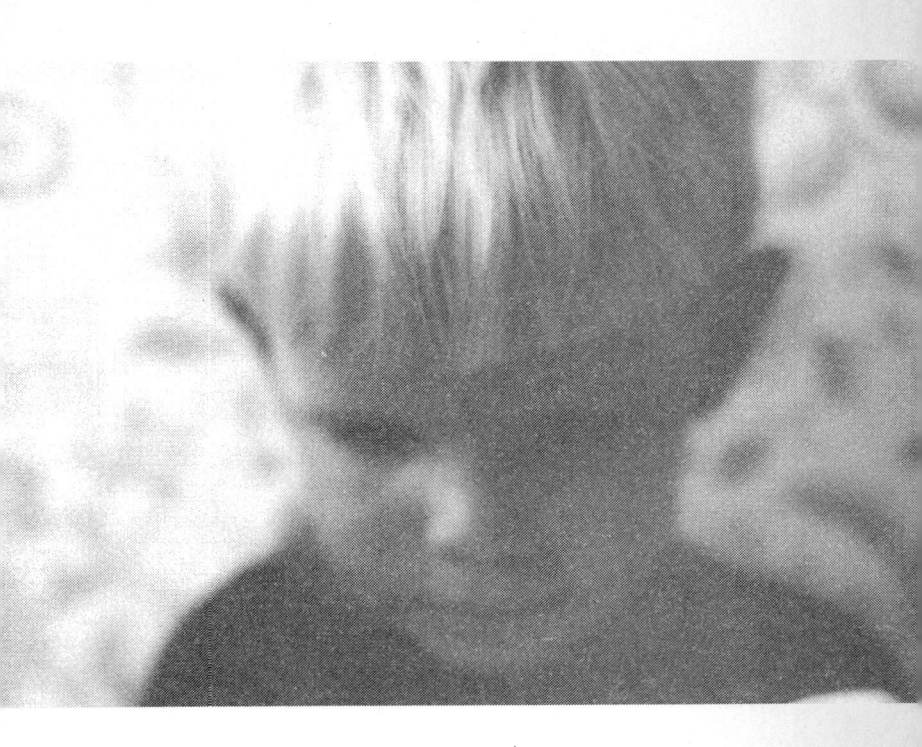

[10]

When Things Go Wrong

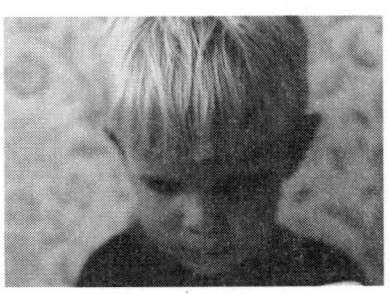

IT'S IN the papers. A boy of eight has been expelled from school and has been caught by the police breaking into an empty house. A group of mothers living in a nearby neighbourhood talk about him at one of their weekly coffee mornings. Diane, the most outspoken, declares that he must have been born that way. She adds that his family are likely to be on the social benefit and are a drain on society. Other mothers agree. They have had no direct contact with abused or neglected children. The lives of these children seem distant and their behaviour inexplicable. The dramatisation of their actions by newspaper articles and TV news is not helpful.

This lack of awareness and of shared concern is a tragedy for this boy and the thousands of others like him. The new evidence on brain development provides an excellent framework for understanding the source of his harm, his misunderstood behaviours, and the need for early action.

Abuse, violence and a chaotic home life

Andy is almost five. He has been referred to a paediatrician because he has witnessed something no one should ever see — his father beating his mother. These 'incidents' stretch back to the time when he had no words to tell. The trauma and the terror have left no visible marks or scars but they have left an imprint on the most important of all his organs — his brain. It is an imprint which has changed his brain's physical structure and chemical balance and carries risks of lifelong disorder if he does not receive swift intervention and effective healing. It is an imprint stamped into his brain-stem, persisting without conscious recognition, and the source of his current behaviour.[1, 2]

Just as the brain adapts to love and nurture, the same is true for violence and abuse. Living in the cross-fire of family violence, Andy's behaviour of being constantly aware and reading unspoken cues is highly adaptive. The ultimate betrayal comes when he moves to other social settings where the same behaviour destroys his learning, his ability to form relationships, and erodes his chances in life.

Early disadvantages

Andy was also found to have been physically abused and neglected. Children like him often, but not exclusively, come from families with many disadvantages. These range from social isolation, unemployment, poverty and the effects of generations of abuse, violence and disorder. They are prone to harm both before and after birth although this is not limited to children from such backgrounds.

Andy's mother was regularly beaten and verbally assaulted during her pregnancy. This resulted in changes in the foetal brain through the exposure to high levels of the hormones and chemicals released under stress. The result was seen in Andy's irritability and difficulty in settling as a baby. His mother lacked the resources to handle this, hindering the development of a bond between them. The result of this struggle was a difficult relationship with Andy from the start. Exposure to toxic substances prior to birth — cannabis, heavy doses of nicotine and alcohol — was also part of his inheritance as it is with many similarly disadvantaged children.

The next problem was intermingled with his mother's impoverished early relationship. Trauma and chaos were also a part of his parents' early lives. Their lack of skills and the emotional capacity to raise children was first witnessed by their lack of consistent, warm and rapid responses to his signals of distress in crying. His mother's responses were unpredictable, often hurtful, and at times he was left unconsoled. His father rarely attended to him. Andy remained hyper-aroused, over-reactive to any stimuli and remained vulnerable to daily stress even to such things as being picked up and handled.

The primary damage

As an infant Andy was wary of his parents, particularly his father. In self-protection, he learned to seek their attention infrequently. They did not demonstrate any warmth towards him but instead ignored him except to feed him, bath him and put him to bed. The daily timetable suited their activities and not his needs. Witnessing and hearing the terrifying sounds of violence became an integral part of his life. Cut off from any attachment, he also developed no sense of internal reward or an understanding of others.

At this early age Andy was already demonstrating the damaging effects of being raised in an abusive and violent home. Driven by fear and terror, his brain's development has been shaped by the persistent activation of the survival response. In this sustained form it has reduced his capacity to process other experiences, has affected his memory and suppressed his immune system. It has also coloured his perception of all else, leaving him to see his entire world as dangerous. Living in fear has also caused his survival response to become more easily sparked and to lead to a more intense arousal of his brain. He survives in a persistent state of anxiety but displays no obvious external sign of this. The hidden markers are a raised pulse and heart rate, a slightly raised temperature and a fast metabolic rate which allows him to eat ravenously but remain skinny. With the increase in the sensitivity of his survival response, triggers hidden in his mind now cause its actions. He has no conscious recognition of them and to others they are also inexplicable. Andy, as a result, is left open to disabling post-traumatic cueing — to being suddenly confronted in his mind with the feelings and emotions evoked by his original source of harm and his father's violence.

The associated behaviours

Andy's mother cannot handle his continued irritability, constant activity, and general lack of attention except to television. Andy is unrestricted in viewing time or the programmes selected. His mother has used television since he was an infant to keep him out of her way. As such, he sees brutal and bloody programmes that reinforce his home experiences. Sadly, this continual trauma leads to a failure of another step in the development of his brain, compounding the effects of this additional violence. His higher brain areas have not developed sufficiently to modulate and regulate some of the lower brain functions — the functions seen in his difficult behaviour that so exhausts his mother. This failure is caused by the overuse of Andy's survival response that has overwhelmed the capacity for any regulation by his higher brain areas. The legacy of this is an unfettered impulsivity and easy arousal. This is what happens to his father who, when drunk, loses the same higher inhibitory control and becomes impulsive and violent.

Now almost five, Andy's current behaviour swings from withdrawal, when he seems unaware of what is going on, to aggression. His aggressive tendencies, displayed when his father is absent, now leave him uncontrollable. His mother had previously frequently assaulted Andy and his brothers, verbally and physically releasing her pain on them when their father was out of the home. She now cannot cope with Andy's aggression and instead verbally abuses or attempts to isolate him — both actions simply making his behaviour worse and not better. Now that he is strong enough, Andy responds by physically attacking his mother during unpredictable episodes of violence and destruction.

The cause of this last devastating set of circumstances for Andy remains hidden. Normally, the survival or stress response requires an external source of threat or danger to trigger it. When this happens the individual moves quickly from calm to fear, returning to normal once the problem has gone. It does not work this way for Andy. His hypersensitive response and constant anxiety allows minor triggers, hidden in his mind, to catapult him instantly to a state of terror. When this happens, access to the cerebral cortex is lost and only the lower brain functions. Andy's sense of time becomes disjointed and he is not aware of the internal interactions that sparked these reactions and why he suddenly felt challenged, angry, fearful or just needed to lash out. His mother's actions only reinforce his view that all adults use power and violence to achieve control. It is a dangerous concept that is already invading his limited ability to solve problems in any other way.

Adaptive to maladaptive

For Andy, raised in an unpredictable, chaotic and violent environment, his brain's reaction to these experiences is highly successful. His brain is hyperviligant and has a sensitive arousal system. Frequently assaulted by his mother, he is quick to act on impulse and strike out before being struck. With his primary relationships characterised by neglect and unreliability, he has learnt that intimacy is to be avoided.

Unfortunately the tragedy for Andy, and all traumatised children, comes through these behaviours. The last downhill slope occurs when they move outside the home to be faced with other adults and children. In a different social setting, their behaviour is no longer appropriate. With most children this comes with school. Whether at school or pre-school these children display behaviour that ranges from persistent hyper-arousal to dissociation. This erodes their chances of integrating successfully and, sadly, they don't recognise what is happening.

In the face of inescapable trauma, infants and toddlers detach themselves from reality through dissociation. Andy cuts his conscious mind in this way from his father's terrorising assaults on his mother and her abuse of him. It also cuts him off from all other experiences, including learning. Such dissociation is caused by the same set of chemicals that calm a baby at birth and dampen arousal, and despite its serious outcomes, it is unlikely to be noticed. When this happens at school he will probably be described as inattentive, dreamy or incapable of learning.

But like many children, he displays behaviour from both ends of the continuum; he becomes hyper-aroused — unpredictably assaulting his mother and erupting into episodes of defiance and difficulty. Such behaviour is more common in boys from a chaotic and uncaring background, and soon brings them to attention at school. Their problems range from sudden outbursts of violence and destruction to a cluster of symptoms, which mimic and are often misdiagnosed as the Attention Deficit Hyperactivity Disorder (ADHD). It is their hyper-arousal, not hyperactivity, that is the driving force. The short attention span, the constant focusing on non-verbal cues, and the bar to the cortex result in an inability to think rationally or listen.

These reactions are reinforced when adults, understandably but inappropriately, confront the child and attempt to control the behaviour. Andy requires work to achieve consistent, predictable relationships and secure environments at home and at school with predictable daily timetables. This is his one opportunity to learn and to heal. It is only through this difficult co-ordinated approach that both his arousal and dissociation can be avoided and his conscious mind engaged. When he is calm he can understand what causes his behaviour when this is discussed with him. This is most helpful. Yet when aroused or dissociating, he reverts to automatic reflexive reactions where this information has no place.

The impact of neglect

Neglect leaves its own trail of destruction in the developing brain, and can be even more difficult to deal with than abusive experiences. The term neglect usually refers to the physical presentation of the child, yet it is the lack of experiences driving development that is actually more dangerous. This is common to all neglect but is rarely recognised or acted upon. Caused by lack of interaction by parents, it has two forms: one when these experiences are denied, and the other when they are unpredictable. The lack or denial of the developmental needs in early childhood provides, at its worst, the ultimate evidence of how experiences shape the growing brain. At its most cruel, this is seen in children whose early lives were spent locked in a room or cupboard or in an emotionally destitute institution. These children have head circumferences well below normal — an accurate measure of brain volume under the age of four. Imaging of their brains graphically shows how the lack of stimulation to the cerebral cortex has impaired its development and growth.

Such disasters may be rare but many neglected children on the same spectrum with less damage are simply not recognised or ignored until too late. They may display delayed intellectual, verbal and social skills as well as a difficulty with attachment. With some children, the related loss of cortical growth and function is mirrored by a corresponding loss of the modulating capacity on lower brain function. In short, they are impulsive, unattached, over-reactive to any stimuli and delayed. They present a draining and difficult combination of behaviour for their parents and other caregivers. These children require work to provide the experiences they have missed. This must centre on their impoverished attachment and their developmental stage, not their age. It is long-term, difficult and often frustrating therapy, but gains can be made.

The other common form of neglect comes with the lack of patterned consistent early experiences and warm, responsive caregiving. These children are raised in households where the parents are unavailable, unwilling, or lack the skills to raise them. Like Andy, they are also often abused. Their brain organisation, attachment and empathy is disordered or lacking. Their symptoms range from the discomfort of mildly impaired inter-personal relationships to profound social and emotional problems. In addition, the dangerous lack of any sense of internal reward and pleasure frequently leads to the adoption of behaviours that are serious risks to their health as they seek to artificially gain their 'highs'. Self-mutilation, glue sniffing, smoking, drugs and alcohol are among the methods used. Such behaviours, combined with the frequent sense of alienation for many who are isolated by family and school, contribute to anti-social and criminal activities, joining gangs, engaging in indiscriminate remorseless violence, and even suicide.

The behaviour of these children or the deficiencies of their families are all too often used as reasons or excuses for taking no action. This failure to intervene early on behalf of these children deepens their disadvantages — the opportunity to act when the brain can still easily compensate and change is lost. The children are robbed of their potential — sometimes their total potential — when there was no reason why, with early assistance they could not have had normal intellectual abilities, full sensory development and healthy attachments.

Poverty and neglect

Poverty, more than any other social factor, can lead to neglect and damages young children's brains. The disadvantages for these families are numerous — the lack of transport or telephone, poor nutrition, poor and crowded housing, a lack of access to or knowledge of childcare and education, and high levels of stress. Some of these children have poor relationships with their parents and are exposed to family violence. They also have few opportunities for stimulation and play. Day-care, if available, is commonly inadequate and crime is often endemic within the local community. This is a real concern in this country with one in three children now estimated to live in poverty.[3]

Studies show that children from economically and socially disadvantaged families are less likely to be prepared for school and their intellectual development is more likely to be delayed. Other studies have detailed how as these children pass through school their learning declines as does their ability to get on with others. They will also have problems regulating their emotions and are a huge demand on special education services. Those children most at risk are those whose homes are chaotic and abusive. The children who thrive despite these disadvantages are those with a strong attachment to their parents. Those parents living in poverty who nevertheless care for their children usually know something about child development, and usually have access to social support and assistance for any of their own issues, especially those relating to abuse or neglect in their own childhood.

The implications

The risks to these children do not need to determine their destiny. Many children have succeeded despite traumatising and neglectful early years. Most were given help or gained the protection of a caring adult outside the home. To alter the present ignorance about the harm these children face requires widespread knowledge and understanding. The implications for current systems are enormous.

The critical element of timing cannot be overplayed. This timing must be based on the astronomical and rapid changes in young children's developing brains. The judge who decides that more physical evidence is needed to remove a two-year-old child from her home and asks for a review in six months is ill-informed. So is the doctor who realises that a three-year-old is being neglected at home but procrastinates and decides to wait until the 'next' visit. Both are inept and dangerous decisions. Six months for a two-year-old child is equivalent to a life sentence for an adult. Several months can permanently impair the brain development of the three-year-old child. Any action must reflect the child's needs, not those of adults, and the emphasis should be the child's safety and recovery, not any potential charge against an offender.

Many thousands of the children referred to the statutory services each year are found to be maltreated. Many of these children are too young to tell. These children are consistently absorbing and adapting to the horrors, and carry the scars into their adolescent and adult lives.

Many studies detail the consequences of pervasive anxiety, depression, conduct disorders, substance abuse and school failure. As they grow, such children are plagued by dependency, violence, criminality, and psychiatric, psychological and psychosomatic problems. As well, a wide range of high health-risk behaviours can be traced to their childhood abuse or neglect, and in turn, to the leading cause of deaths in adults — cancer, stroke, AIDS, liver, lung and heart disease.[4] Added to this are the risks of replicating the same damage in their own children.

The consequences are so diverse that, like a braided river, their shared beginning is not recognised while the ever-escalating costs of attempting to control or contain the individual problems are beyond the resources of many countries. The losses include the loss of human potential. These children either turn their pain inwards or pass it on to others in destructive ways. In so doing, they are robbing society of their unrealised potential and eroding the security, success and humanity of the nation as a whole.

Hurt and troubled children need early recognition, early intervention, a comprehensive assessment and individual planned healing. We need to instigate the cost-effective systems seen in other countries to prevent this damage. The result of failure to do this — a legacy of children who are impulsive, fearful, aggressive or silently destroyed — is intolerable when the answers are known.

Fact file

- Neglect or abuse can impair or destroy the development of the brain leading to disastrous results for children. These range from those children who can neither tolerate nor learn from normal daily stress to those whose early life experiences leave a legacy of anti-social or self-destructive behaviour.

- Abused children living in violent or chaotic homes are unable to learn, lack social skills, and are at risk of developing other damaging behaviour with lifelong consequences. This has been widely documented in children who witness or hear such violence between their parents without any personal physical injury.

- The behaviour of abused children is often not amenable to traditional forms of therapy based on information and reason.

- The two forms of developmental neglect have serious consequences including an interference with basic skills and abilities and the loss or disorder of attachment. These results are due to the lack of growth of related brain networks.

Things to do
For parents and childcare, early education and health workers

- If you are worried about a child, particularly one not yet at school, seek advice or report the child to a statutory service or some other professional who can help. Ensure that you are informed about what has happened to the child after reporting.

- That advice may initially come from someone you know who works in this field — someone within a statutory service or health workers such as general practitioners.

- If you remain concerned and unsatisfied with any result, seek advice again or re-report the family — specifying any continued or new concerns.

- Never label a child with their behaviours or attribute their failure as inevitable because of their family. Look for the causes behind their presentations.

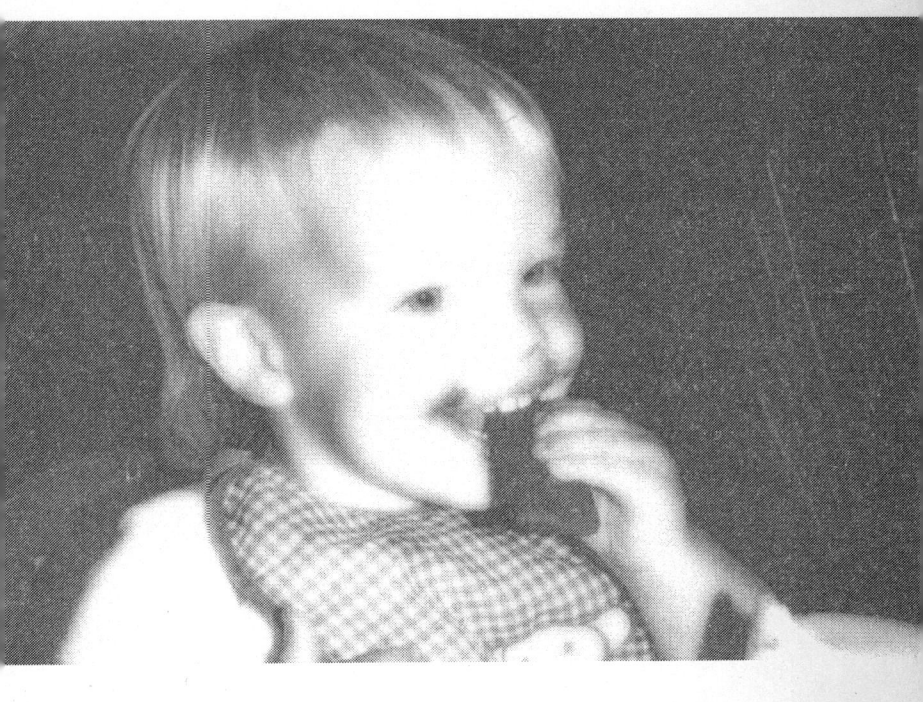

[11]

Nutrition, the Brain and Health

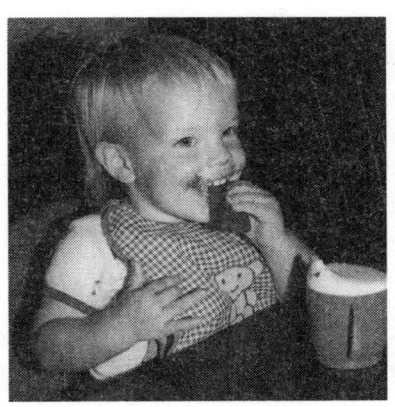

THE BRAIN controls the body. Does it in any way influence health throughout life? Conversely, does a baby's nutrition have any impact on the brain's development and its workings? While babies do have an essential source of brain development in their nurture and care, does anything else matter? The answers are incomplete but compelling.

Before birth

Before birth and continuing into the second year of life the brain is an immensely active organ. It demands 20 per cent of the body's total oxygen supply and steady levels of glucose. During this time protein deficiencies can lead to disturbances in the production of essential neurotransmitters, and iron deficiency can cause later short attention spans, impaired memory and difficulties in learning. Poor nutrition in foetal life has also been linked to later coronary heart disease, hypertension and diabetes.[1]

By birth the active brain is ready to take on the challenges of the world. For this brain to be healthy, the mother must have had a well-balanced diet and avoided smoking, alcohol and drugs to reduce the associated risks to the brain and the related risks of a pre-term birth or a low-birth-weight baby. Any physical and emotional trauma in pregnancy can also cause disturbed functioning of the foetal and the new-born's brain.

Milk: the first nutrition

Feeding a baby provides both the nutrition of the essential ingredients in milk and the essential requirements of nurture and touch. These are significant, related influences on brain development and later behaviour. As it is, nurturing tends to be more important than nutrition and the brain's development is not necessarily impaired by poor nutrition if the baby's experiences are stimulating, challenging, consistent and nurturing.[2,3]

Breast-feeding has been shown to provide both optimal nutrition and stimulation for new-born babies and infants. This is hardly surprising — this is nature at work. The act of breast-feeding brings many sensory experiences for both the mother and the child. In addition, breast milk provides a more balanced, complete diet than formula milk, which has been identified as lacking two elements that could possibly affect the forming brain. These are iron and two specific forms of polyunsaturated fatty acids. These two types of fatty acids are found in small amounts in breast milk but are absent from cow's milk, the milk used in making the majority of formulas. The eye and the brain are rich in both of these components. Pre-term and low-birth-weight babies seem to need at least one of these fats, although term babies need neither. A number of studies have been undertaken to see whether fortifying or supplementing formula milk can promote development in term and pre-term infants. To date, there has been no clear answer. Similarly, it is still unclear whether part of the advantage for cognitive development of breast-fed babies is enhanced by these polyunsaturated fatty acids.

Iron deficiency, inevitable for children living in impoverished countries, is also a silent enemy for many living in affluent nations. Anaemia is the last sign to appear. Among the first symptoms are irritability and a general unwellness. It continues with a high sensitivity to infection, poor physical growth, a decrease of muscular strength and a lack of energy. Those symptoms interfere with children's ability to explore and learn. Among infants and children, it can also lead to delayed mental and motor development.

The influence of sensory experiences

Breast-feeding is not an option for many mothers, particularly if they work outside the home or lack assistance to establish the process. Nevertheless, there is evidence that breast-feeding stimulates physical and mental development. Breast-fed children have been shown to perform better in tests that assess their cognitive development, verbal ability and school performance. However, these findings are influenced by two factors. The first involves the very intimate act of breast-feeding. Simply embracing the baby while feeding provides opportunities for multiple sensory experiences — skin-to-skin contact, visual contact, the mother's voice and the smell of her body and of the milk. Touch is a key stimulus to brain development at this stage in life. Where breast-feeding is not possible, bottle-feeding should involve the same holding, cuddling and talking to the baby.

The second factor is that mothers in these studies over the past few decades tend to come from higher socio-economic groups. Their babies obviously benefit from higher parental education, better nutrition and housing, a more stimulating environment and access to pre-school education. When these advantages are taken into account, however, most of these studies still suggest that there are distinct advantages to breast-feeding.

The message for mothers who have no choice but to bottle-feed is to ensure that their children enjoy the same sensory experiences while feeding.

Poor nutrition

Disasters, wars and famines have wreaked havoc on the food available to children across the centuries, particularly in the Third World. Some of this devastation is now seen in inner city ghettos and neglected populations in affluent countries. Subtler threats to brain development are also increasing in these nations where undernourished children appear physically normal but their intellectual development is impaired. These young children go to pre-school or school without breakfast, bring no lunch and are chronically underfed at home. They are tired, less active, more apathetic and disinterested in their surroundings. They will be socially withdrawn, lack curiosity and the drive to learn. A poor iron intake is common, adding to their lethargy, their lack of attention and their inability to concentrate or remember.

Fortunately, programmes that deliver breakfast to children and supplementary food to women and infants have been shown to have positive effects on their cognitive development. These benefits include higher performance on standardised tests, better school attendance, lowered incidence of anaemia and a reduced need for expensive special education. There is additional evidence that child development programmes started in early life and involving parents can influence how they relate to and care for their children. The long-term effects include vast improvements in the children's learning, behaviour and health in later life with the benefits seen in children from all social and economic backgrounds.

The brain and physical health

Anja was a placid, happy toddler until her father left home in what was a bitter, divisive and at times violent divorce. Subsequently, her mother allowed another partner to move into the home. There are suggestions that the step-father at times abused Anja. Whatever happened to the child left no marks and was never named. As she grew she became withdrawn as a little girl and was bullied at school. The ups and downs of her behaviour finally deteriorated when she joined a group of children known to be disruptive and difficult. As a teenager she would accept no help and spoke to no one about her feelings. Now she is 20 and both her body and her mind are affected. She is depressed, isolated, seems to be constantly unwell and, after bouts of acute abdominal pain and diarrhoea with bleeding, she has been found to have colitis.

What had happened? The possible fear and terror of her parents' divorce may have harmed her forming brain together with the likely loss of her mother's attention and affection. Perhaps if her mother had been able to nurture Anja through that difficult time, the outcome would have been different. Other possible factors include the way her sensory experiences in her early life helped shape her brain's endocrine and immune pathways.[4]

The endocrine system controls the release of hormones, a major communication system in the body. There is a combined central control for the release of key hormones that act on organs with the capacity to release others into the blood. These act on target tissues and the brain. It is a system that is vital for activating basic behavioural activities such as sex, emotion, stress and the regulation of body functions such as growth, energy use and metabolism. The immune system controls the cells that fight infection and other foreign material in the body. The autonomic nervous system conserves or releases energy and resources depending on the presence or absence of a threat or danger.

Threatened or stressed, the brain will activate these systems. The immune system responds by redistributing its cells to their battle stations. One section of the autonomic system redirects blood to the muscles and increases the heart rate and blood pressure. The stress hormones, adrenaline and cortisol, are released. Adrenaline puts the body into a state of arousal, while cortisol mobilises energy by increasing the glucose available to the muscles and later helping the body to recover. Once the danger has passed, these responses dissipate.

Persistent or chronic stress, such as the trauma faced by Anja as a child, damages the function of these systems and the brain. When high levels of the hormones are released over a long period, they affect and disrupt the memory of the events surrounding the trauma. Persistent stress can also cause a loss of brain cells in the organ of the brain responsible for these memories. Over time, cortisol and adrenaline together contribute to physical ill health, leading to high blood pressure, abdominal obesity, hardening of the arteries as well as other stress-associated physical disorders. Colitis is included in this list. Under repeated stress, the immune system can be inhibited, bringing a vulnerability to infections. This is the probable underlying cause of Anja's constant illnesses. Isolated, without support and lacking coping skills, she may suffer from another loss. Scientists are investigating how a sense of helplessness can eventually diminish the long-term effectiveness of the immune system.

We are only now beginning to understand the biological pathways through which the brain influences health. It is an evolving frontier but when combined with the social factors affecting health, such research is likely to show how brain development and function can alter health risks throughout the life cycle.

The brain and mental health

Anja is likely to suffer from other problems. We already know that a history of abuse and trauma can permanently damage the forming brain, resulting in a wide range of mental and psychological disorders. However, there is another extraordinary component to this unfolding story. The implications are profound. They describe the normal daily working of the brain which, when out of order, is capable of determining the mental health even of those whose childhood was not traumatic or violent.

The story began 65 years ago with the detection of neurotransmitters — the chemicals that assist the transport of the brain cell messages. Next came the knowledge of how they worked. More recently there has been an explosion of information about their wide effects on the body and the mind. We are also discovering far more of these neurotransmitters. Originally only two were discovered but now 100 have been identified and this is likely to double. These neurotransmitters are similar to certain plant products such as opium that for centuries have been used to alter moods and consciousness. Understanding how these neurotransmitters work should help explain the biological basis of mental illness and the circuits responsible for some devastating brain disorders.

Neurotransmitters have a wide range of functions. Endorphins, for example, are potent natural painkillers, known to give a high to long distance runners and athletes. Their structure is similar to morphine. Another chemical is involved with the action of voluntary muscles and may be critical in the functioning of normal attention and memory. Two other linked chemicals play a role in movement, the regulation of hormones, learning and psychiatric disorders such as schizophrenia. Another chemical has been found to influence consciousness, mood, depression and anxiety as well as the regulation of violence.

Researchers have also recently found separate systems of chemicals in the brain that are necessary for the development, function and survival of certain groups of brain cells. A greater understanding of these neurotransmitters and chemicals required by the brain will allow the design of medications to specifically address some of the effects of mental illnesses and degenerative and developmental neural disorders. The story of these amazing chemicals, the story of one avenue through which the brain affects the mind and the body, is set to continue.

Fact file

- Good maternal nutrition during pregnancy, including a diet with adequate folic acid and iron, is essential for the baby to develop a healthy brain.
- Feeding provides a baby with both nutrition and sensory stimulus. For this reason breast milk is preferable to formulas.
- Iron deficiency in children can cause delays in motor and mental development and a wide range of other problems that affect learning.
- Poorly nourished children are less active and are disinterested, reducing their natural curiosity and drive to learn.
- Chronic or persistent stress can affect the developing brain and the immune system as well as causing later physical diseases.
- Neurotransmitters affect a wide range of moods, emotions and behaviour, including violence and psychiatric disorders.

Things to do

For parents

- Pay attention to diet during pregnancy and the nutrition of babies and young children to help ensure good brain development.
- If bottle-feeding, remember to hold, cuddle and embrace the child in the same way you would if breast-feeding.
- If you have any worries about whether your baby's or child's nutrition is adequate ask a dietician.

For childcare, health and early education workers

- If you work in a pre-school or a day-care centre with poorly nourished children ask a community service to provide the food they need. You should also bring this to the attention of the public health and welfare systems in your area. Some of their families will need assistance on many levels.

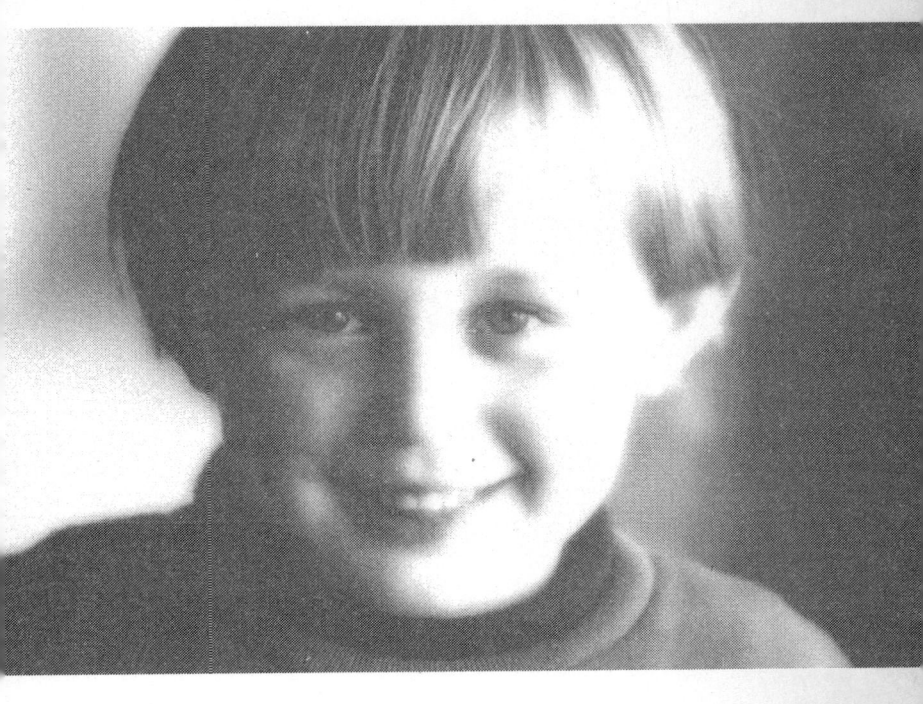

[12]

Personality and Temperament

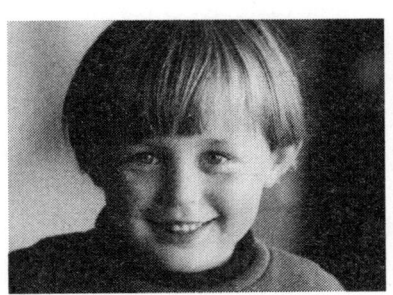

PERSONALITY IS usually defined as a combination of temperament and learned experience. Temperament, on the other hand, is usually defined as the individual character that permanently affects the manner of acting, thinking and feeling. These issues are highlighted with Denise's daughter, Moana. At six months she has her aunt Julia's outgoing and happy temperament. Other relatives agree. It must be the genes. Her aunt is successful and everyone hopes that Moana, with a similar inheritance, will be too. Christine, the next door neighbours' child, is a year old but has not been so lucky. She is excessively shy. The general consensus is that her genes will inevitably bring her problems as she grows.

Is this assumption correct? How much does a child's genetic inheritance contribute to her personality and temperament? How much do her experiences and the environment alter this directive? All the answers are not available but it is becoming clear that while a tendency to some characteristics may be genetically determined, this never defines a child's destiny. Genetics may provide the basic messages but the experiences of life determine the ultimate expression of these individual orientations to the world.

Changing the direction

So how much is personality defined by temperament? Let's look at Christine, Moana's next door neighbour, as she grows up. As a toddler she was so shy that she found it difficult to play with other children and impossible to leave her parents when she was out. At pre-school this became a real barrier to her social development. Her parents sought help and luckily the advice they were given was the answer. With her mother present she attended a programme of music and movement classes and learnt to enjoy her body, the music, and the children. Coaxed by her mother, she and Moana regularly played together. Gaining in self-confidence, she made friends when she entered school and was able to participate in all the activities of her class. By six she was a happy, bubbly child.

An inherited tendency to shyness was undoubtedly part of Christine's personality. This is one of several genes or familial vulnerabilities that scientists have identified that seem to carry a variety of emotional behaviours, from risk taking and aggressiveness to happiness. But it is not so simple. As in other areas of the brain's development, genes and any inherited tendency act in partnership with the experiences of children. A shy infant or aggressive child treated with love and trust can change their behaviour and defy their genetic blueprint. A gene is only a tendency to a trait — not a guarantee. For that trait to be realised, the gene must be switched on by environmental factors. The environment can alter genetic predilections.

Changing an inherited tendency, even one that seems to predict future problems for the child, can expose hidden talents. One such example is risk-taking, which has been connected to a disorder of the receptors for a particular neurotransmitter. This leaves the child less sensitive to pain and physical sensations. Ken was one such child. A source of continual anxiety for his parents, he used to climb, crash, and hurt himself to see what the feelings were like. His bruises, stitches and scars were sources of pride he displayed to other children. Yet his dominance over his peers left him with no friends. His parents realised that he needed special attention to avoid this behaviour escalating to aggression and bullying. They identified the goals. Ken was given the extra warmth and nurture he required. They ensured he had friends to play with and from this he learnt co-operative forms of behaviour and shared his toys with others. Agreed limits were firm but given with understanding to instil a control of his assertiveness. Games that he liked were used to redirect his energy, and rules protecting others were strictly applied. In conversation he was encouraged to identify his own feelings and consider his own needs. Simply talking about the consequences of his actions helped him develop a consideration of others. Treated with this early understanding and support, Ken grew to become an imaginative and enterprising leader in his adolescence.

Negative and positive interactions

Some traits or behaviour make it more predictable as to the way a baby may be handled.[1] Terry was a baby who was 'colicky', irritable and slow to smile. He also slept poorly. His parents, unable to find a solution, began to blame each other and became more negative and detached when interacting with him. In this way, from the outset Terry was labelled as difficult and unresponsive. Yet there may have been many underlying causes. A pain associated with feeding? An allergy to his milk? A tendency to be more sensitive to touch or to sound? In contrast, his older brother, Richard, had an ideal start. From the beginning he was happy, interactive and eagerly seeking his parents' attention. In return he was hugged, caressed and endorsed. His outgoing disposition has reinforced these elements, so that now at eight he is confident and optimistic.

These two babies in part determined the relationship each had with the same parents. This has important implications for disadvantaged babies like Terry. What is crucial is that any inherited tendencies or physical reactions do not limit or define a child's potential or the way parents respond to that child. Negative patterns of interaction are often very difficult to change once established. It is only by comprehensively assessing the baby's behaviour and symptoms, and how the parents respond, that solutions can be found. Terry was found to have reflux, the milk and gastric juices burning the area of the inlet to his stomach, and an intense sensitivity to sound. With proper medical attention to both these problems, there was a dramatic response in the handling and the warmth he received. As importantly, his brain's development was no longer threatened by the unintentional neglect and intrusive actions of his parents. Terry, now three, remains an active, easily overloaded child but one whose parents understand him.

Fact file

- The individual differences of babies and infants can result from inherited tendencies and pre-natal influences. Yet like all behaviour and dispositions they can be altered by their experiences.

- Future research will identify more about the changes in brain development that may be associated with any related tendency. This will give the opportunity to examine any beneficial treatment.

- Negative patterns of interaction are often difficult to change once established. The underlying causes need to be assessed and patterns of behaviour modified.

Personality and Temperament

Things to do

For parents and all childcare workers

- Seek assistance early if you or someone you know are having difficulties responding to your baby or young child.

- Try to identify the needs of the child as well as the parents' or your own needs when seeking help.

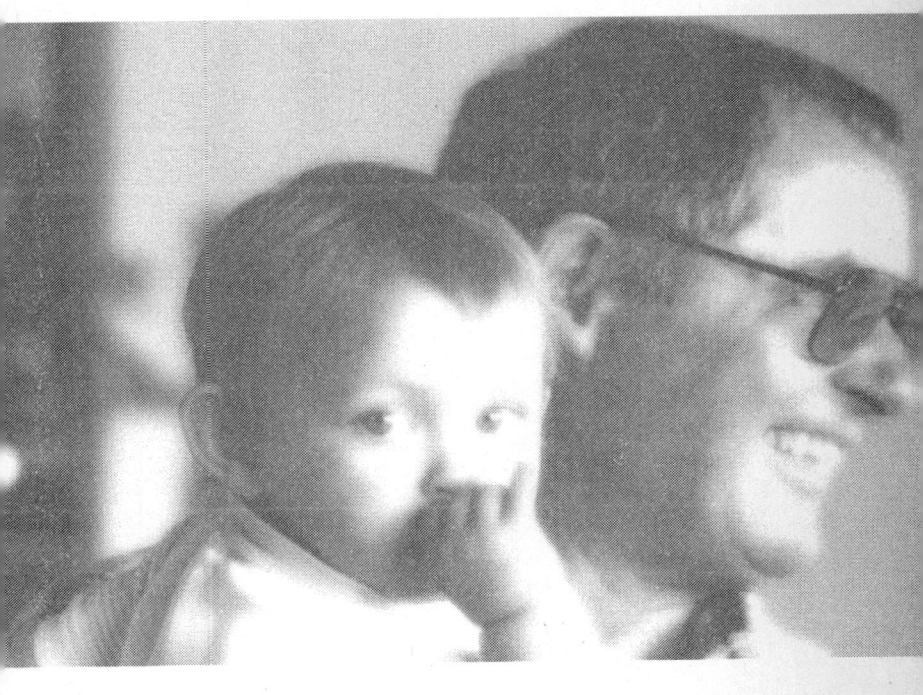

[13]

The Challenge

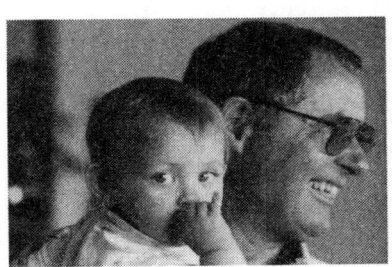

A BABY CRIES, an infant demands, a toddler asserts himself. All require a large amount of time and attention to provide the intimate care and rich emotional experiences needed if their minds are to grow. Time will need to be spent sharing their interests, following their curiosity, and doing things they enjoy. Their intellect, their potential skills and abilities, their health and, above all, their capacity to care for others will depend on this attention.

The difficulties in providing this care have become insurmountable for too many parents. The later costs — to the children, to families and to the nation — are enormous. If left unattended this country will continue on a downhill slide as the under-educated, poorly skilled, and violent members of society inflict their damage.

Can you do any more than care for your own children or those you work with? It is worth looking at the current barriers as well as the option of sharing a commitment to improve the lives of young children.

The barriers

The erosion of the care and concern for children in recent years has been dramatic. This erosion stems partly from families, partly from within communities, as well as resulting from national and global preoccupations. All are linked with one thread running through them all: a materialistic and self-promoting vision of life that disregards the compassion, nurture and safety necessary for human survival and essential to the blossoming of the potential of every child.

Global trends have led to sweeping changes in the world's economic systems with huge multinational corporations that lack humane concerns. Similarly, the instant, invisible transfer of money has collectively destroyed the older, slower and more insightful systems under the control of individual countries. These changes have undermined the ability of some nations to manage their resources and can destroy the lives of entire populations. This powerful technological revolution has an historical equivalent in the Industrial Revolution which also caused a wide and disturbing disruption of economies and social circumstances.

The national response to these changes has included the withdrawal of social responsibility by the State, the pursuit of a free-market economy with its adverse implications for the disadvantaged, the promotion of personal enterprise, adult privacy, competitiveness and the expansion of a faceless bureaucracy. The effects, in just 16 years, have changed this country from one with little inequality to a country with a canyon between the rich and the poor.[1] We now know that under these circumstances, the health risks of those at the bottom of the pile is increased substantially.[2] This divide in wealth and poverty has, in turn, led to an increase in violent crime by those impoverished and alienated. At the other end, indulged materialistic children, with the same empty emotional lives as their disadvantaged counterparts, wreak similar damage when they eventually assume positions of power. These disasters have been avoided in some countries.[3, 4] Others that have shared the same consequences are actively putting in place opportunities to turn this around.[5] These changes are based on improving the lives of disadvantaged families and their children — armed with the knowledge of the critical importance of the first years of life.

Local communities have also suffered. They are now expected to provide many services discarded by governments without giving the resources, training or money. The diminished funding excludes any co-operation and sharing. Public health and welfare services are often more preoccupied with funding issues than providing essential support and services to the children and families in their communities.

The family itself is under threat. In recent years its basic structure has disintegrated with single-parent family units now increasingly the norm. Parents now not only have to hold down a job but raise their children by themselves, without support or financial security. They are often too tired, too busy or preoccupied to give their children the time and the attention they require.

If this were not enough there are other forces that are equally destructive to early childhood development. As individuals within society we are becoming more isolated. Isolation destroys communities, families and children — destroying the close relationships that define how children learn. The Internet can provide access to pornographic and abusive material, and the means to live our lives without any social interaction. The dominance of television has destroyed social exchange within many families. How is the barrage of violent imagery on television affecting the minds of children? We have become a nation of couch potatoes — increasingly inactive and obese, a time bomb counting down to later related diseases.

The disregard of early childhood is seen in its most dramatic form by looking at the resources and investments made throughout the human lifecycle. In health, education, income support and social services, the critical early years are ignored. These are the years when we can do infinitely more than at any other age to ensure success in life. These are the years which offer the chance to diminish the escalating costs of later disorders, diseases, violence and crime.

What can be done

Strong action is needed if this country and the next generation are to be rescued. We need a change in public understanding and a collective commitment. This commitment involves the courage to stand by our children and challenge the current course and conscience of this nation.

The place to begin is with ourselves. We must ensure that our own children are raised with the care and time they need. We need to spread this message to others and, if possible, help children where that help may be required — a disadvantaged family, a local service, or through a national organisation advocating the needs of early childhood. If time is not available then donate money to an organisation providing for children. At a national level we need to commission a nation-wide study, like those completed elsewhere, analysing in depth all the issues, and devising solutions.

Children cannot wait. This was most eloquently expressed by the Principle of First Call from the 1990 World Summit on Children:[6]

> *That children's one chance of normal development*
> *should receive the first call on all*
> *our concerns and capabilities.*

APPENDIX

New Concepts and Horizons

THE SCIENTIFIC discoveries revealing how the human brain forms have confirmed established observations as well as creating new concepts and dreams. Although for centuries the brain was thought to be an organ of 'minor importance', recent scientific discoveries have highlighted its central place, infinite power and the vast expanses of the mysteries yet to be revealed.

This dramatic leap has a parallel in the exploration of the wonders of space, the stars and the galaxies. The opportunities to study these areas opened by new technologies have exposed unseen worlds and previously undiscovered horizons.

Before birth

Today many women know that their baby is growing well before birth by ultrasound measurements of the baby's head. Ultrasound is now also being used to examine many other organs. A technique developed 20 years ago, this computerised imaging captures the echoes of sound waves bounced off internal organs. Refined with high-resolution recordings, it allows scientists to study brain development before birth. Other developments in embryo transplants, the pre-natal treatment of foetal abnormalities, and imaging tiny preserved slices of the brain at various times of gestation have added to these successes. With these perspectives, the pre-natal development of the brain has been defined as an integral part of its creation.

The examination of brain cells and their connections

For years the major source of knowledge about the internal world of the brain has been through findings at autopsy and the microscopic examination of preserved brain tissues. Recent technical advances have enabled vast increases in the power of the microscopic vision available and an array of techniques to display the cell connections as they develop over time. We also now have different ways of imaging thin slices of brain tissue with techniques to identify specific sites where the necessary chemicals for brain activity become attached. These and other advances have allowed us to determine how some brain cells function, how they reach their precise location, and how networks are formed.

CT scans

The need for greater detail of soft tissues led to the development of Computerised Axial Tomography (CT scans) in the 1970s. Over time there have been continued improvements with these so that they are now a routine part of clinical practice. CT scans are basically X-rays taken in a series of sections and passed to a sensor connected to a computer. This then assembles the images into a comprehensive picture of the brain. When a special dye is injected into a vein, the patterns of the supportive vessels are seen. It is an invaluable tool to investigate the anatomical properties of the brain and its vascular supply — although it cannot demonstrate the brain's function.

Adding the measurement of function

Mapping the function of the brain was resolved by the development of techniques measuring two different aspects of brain activity. One captures the brain's use of energy to show *where* a task is occurring in the brain. The other shows *when* this activity is occurring by measuring the electrical activity of the brain.

Two particular tools, Functional Magnetic Resonance Imaging and Positron Emission Tomography, show *where* a task is occurring in the brain. The gains have been fascinating. Studies have followed specific areas of brain development to show, for example, the emergence of language or to identify the different areas involved in tasks as similar as saying or reading words. Repeated over time these techniques demonstrate the growth of these areas as young children acquire the matched skills and knowledge.

Two other tools are used to map *when* brain activity is occurring — the Electroencephalogram (EEG) and the Event-Related Potential (ERP). These study cognitive and emotional development, especially ERP, which has an excellent resolution in relation to the time of an event being examined.

Functional Magnetic Resonance Imaging (FMRI)

This is one of the most rapidly growing methods used to image the living brain. Producing high-quality 3D images, FMRI scans offer insights into how parts of the brain work. This technique gives information about changes to the volume, flow and oxygenation of the blood as a task is undertaken. These activities can be physical or cognitive, such as speaking or thinking, with the changes seen in the related areas. It requires the person being examined to lie in a large cylindrical magnet as the energy that bounces off atoms in the body is measured. The images are then translated by computers.

This tool has given tremendous insight into the relationship between brain structure and function in adults and is being increasingly used with children. Although non-invasive, it does require that the child lie still in a confined environment and tolerate a relatively high level of noise.

Positron Emission Tomography (PET)

PET is another diagnostic tool linked to the metabolism of the brain. It uses a form of biological mimicry that works through labelling either oxygen or glucose with a radioactive substance. In tricking the brain to use one of these isotopes to drive its activities, the isotopes become concentrated in those areas of the brain which are functioning. A special sensor in the scanner then detects the emitted particles, called positrons, to construct a picture and localise the activity.

This allows scientists to see not only the brain's structure and function but how it uses energy as a variety of tasks are undertaken. Blood flow, oxygen utilisation, protein synthesis and the release of specific systems of chemicals involved can also be measured. The end result is a 3D image reflecting the metabolic and chemical functioning of the brain. Its disadvantages are that it uses radioactivity and is very expensive equipment. It is also unable to define the precise site of an activity beyond a centimetre, or its precise time.

Electroencephalogram (EEG)

The electroencephalogram (EEG) detects and records the background electrical activity of the brain, the 'brain waves', the by-product of the brain cells' communication. Four types of brain waves are associated with different parts of the brain and with different states of activity — from being alert to deep sleep or coma.

It is non-invasive and relatively inexpensive and lends itself to the study of social and emotional development. Because it doesn't cause any discomfort, it can be used to monitor babies and small children. Scientists are using this tool to study how the brain reacts to various external influences such as stress or comfort. In addition, by correlating readings with videotapes of the children engaged in a variety of activities, scientists are able to draw conclusions about the effects of these events on the brain's electrical activity.

Event-Related Potential (ERP)

Electrodes attached to the scalp also record the ERP. The difference from EEG is that it provides excellent resolution in time and can take rapid and repeated records without the child under study needing to respond by speaking or moving. This has allowed it to be used to study cognitive abilities in infants and children such as attention, memory and the comprehension of language.

Analysing chemicals

Other significant techniques for studying brain development and function have come from incredible advances in the analysis of important chemicals and hormones. An example is cortisol, a steroid hormone that rises in stress, and which can now be measured in the saliva. Such measurements give a gauge of the impact of adverse conditions on the brain's biochemistry.

Other major systems of chemicals assist in the transmission of information within the brain. Some of these neurotransmitters have other effects — one is associated in high levels with aggression, and in low levels with autistic disorders.

In hand with the impressive gains in genetics, new techniques have been developed to study the genetic defects which affect the production of these and other chemicals needed for normal brain function. An offshoot of knowledge about the composition of these chemicals and hormones has brought better and more accurate designs for medications aimed at assisting problems originating in the brain.

Gene functioning

Our understanding of genetics has exploded over recent years. Our genes are the inherited message for all human characteristics — short sections of the tightly coiled structures in the nucleus of every cell. These thread-like coils are made of DNA, Deoxyribonucleic Acid, and form the 23 pairs of chromosomes.

Already mapping the more than 100,000 genes contained within each cell has produced answers to many questions — including the early diagnosis of some disorders through pre-natal testing. For example, a common inherited intellectual disability, Fragile X Syndrome, has been identified this way. We are rapidly discovering the entire gene population. This human 'genome' as it is called contains all the biochemical instructions for making and maintaining a human being. With these advances come an immeasurable array of possibilities, many as yet in the realm of dreams.

As more evidence emerges of the interplay between genes and the environment in the development of the brain, we are able to delineate some of the associated problems. For example, some conditions, such as schizophrenia, have an underlying genetic tendency which is only expressed under specific environmental influences. Similarly, environmental factors can sometimes determine how a single gene disorder is expressed. These investigations should help determine controlling influences that contribute to the onset of particular diseases.

GLOSSARY

Adrenaline: A hormone secreted by the adrenal gland affecting the circulation and muscular action.

Autonomic nervous system: A part of the nervous system in the body responsible for regulating the internal organs, particularly in response to stress.

Axon: The long tentacle-like extension of a brain cell through which it sends information to other cells.

Brain-stem: The area of the brain that houses the survival system and controls the vital functions of respiration, heartbeat and blood pressure. It is also the major route through which the higher levels of the brain send and receive information from and to the spinal cord and the peripheral nerves.

Cerebellum: A large convoluted structure above the brain-stem concerned with motor co-ordination.

Cerebral cortex: The outermost layer of the cerebral hemispheres of the brain. It is responsible for all forms of conscious experience including perception, emotion, thought and planning.

Cerebral hemispheres: The two specialised halves of the brain. The left is specialised for speech, writing, language and calculation; the right for spatial recognition, face recognition and some aspects of music perception and production.

Cognition: The process or processes by which an organism gains knowledge of or becomes aware of events or objects in its environment, and uses that knowledge for comprehension and problem solving.

Connection: A gap between two brain cells that functions as the site of information transfer from one to another. (The scientific name is a synapse.)

Cortisol: A hormone manufactured in the adrenal gland. In humans it is secreted in greatest quantities before dawn, readying the body for the activities of the coming day.

Dissociation: The mental process of disengaging from the external environment and attending to the inner. This is a graded process that ranges from daydreaming to pathological disturbance and may include an exclusive focus on an inner fantasy world, loss of identity, disorientation, perceptual disturbances and even disruptions in identity.

Evoked potentials: A measure of the brain's electrical activity in response to sensory stimuli.

Explicit memory: The final phase of memory in which information storage may last from hours to a lifetime (also known as long-term memory).

Glossary

Frontal lobe: One of the four divisions of each hemisphere. Its role is in controlling movement and associating the functions of other cortical areas.

Gene: The biological unit of heredity with each located at a definite position on a particular chromosome.

Hippocampus: A structure in the limbic system with functions in learning, memory and emotion.

Hormones: Chemical messengers secreted by endocrine glands to regulate the activity of target cells. They play a role in sexual development, calcium and bone metabolism, growth and many other activities.

Hyperarousal: Mental and physical changes caused by alterations in the activity of the central and peripheral nervous system in response to a perceived or actual threat. This graded response includes increased sensory and perceptual focus on the threat, the triggering of the physiological systems required for survival, and corresponding changes in emotional and behavioural functioning.

Hypervigilance: The state of increased arousal and attention to any cue in the external environment that may potentially be associated with threat.

Hypothalamus: A small complex brain structure near the base of the brain that regulates such functions as hormonal activity, thirst, hunger, temperature, sex and sleep.

Implicit memory: The memory of abilities that requires no conscious recall.

Limbic system: A group of brain structures that work to help regulate emotion, memory, sexual behaviour, attachment and certain aspects of movement.

Myelin: A compact fatty material that surrounds and insulates the axons of some brain cells.

Neuron: A nerve or brain cell. It is specialised for the transmission of information through axons and short receiving projections.

Neurotransmitter: A chemical released by a neuron to assist the passage of its messages in electrical signals across the connections made with other neurons.

Parietal lobe: One of the four subdivisions of the cerebral cortex. It plays a role in sensory processes, attention and language.

Peripheral nervous system: A division of the nervous system consisting of all nerves not part of the brain or the spinal cord.

Stress: Any challenge or condition that forces the regulating physiological and neurophysiological systems to move outside their normal activity.

Temporal lobe: One of the four subdivisions of the cerebral cortex. It functions in auditory perception, speech and complex visual perceptions.

Thalamus: A structure that is the key relay station for sensory information flowing into the brain, filtering out only information of particular importance from the mass of signals entering the brain.

Trauma: A psychologically distressing event that is outside the range of usual human experience, often involving a sense of intense fear, terror and helplessness.

Working memory: A phase of memory in which a limited amount of information may be held for several seconds to minutes (also known as short-term memory).

REFERENCES

Introduction

1 Shore, R., *Rethinking the Brain: New Insights into Early Development*, Families and Work Institute, New York, 1997.

Chapter 2 Wonderful Parents

1 Gunnar, M. R., *Quality of Care and the Buffering of Stress Physiology: Its Potential Role in Protecting the Developing Human Brain*, University of Minnesota: Institute of Child Development, 1996.

2 Terr, L., 'What happens to early memories of trauma? A study of twenty children under age five at the time of documented traumatic events', *Journal of the American Academy of Child and Adolescent Psychiatry*, Vol. 27, pp. 96–104, 1988.

Chapter 3 The World Begins

1 Scott T. and T. Grice, 'The great brain robbery', The Publishing Trust, Wellington, New Zealand, 1996.

2 Shore R., *Rethinking the Brain: New Insights into Early Development*, Families and Work Institute, New York, 1997.

3 Glass, M., Dragunow, M. and R. L. M. Faull, 'Cannabinoid receptors in the human brain: A detailed anatomical and quantitative autoradiographic study in the fetal, neonatal and adult human brain', *Neuroscience*, Vol. 77, pp. 299–318, 1997.

Chapter 4 Potential and Experiences

1 Nash, J.M., 'Fertile minds', *Time*, 3 February, 1997.

2 Als, H., Lawhon, G., Duffy, F. H., McAnulty, G. B., Gibes-Grossman, R. and J. G. Blickman, 'Individualized developmental care for the very low-birth-weight pre-term infant: Medical and neurofunctional effects', *Journal of American Medical Association*, Vol. 272, pp. 853–58, 1994.

Chapter 5 Movement and Music

1 Prechtl, H. F. R., 'The importance of fetal movements', *Neurophysiology and Neuropsychology of Motor Development*, Connolly, K. J. and H. Forssberg (eds.), Mac Keith Press, Cambridge, 1997.

2 Carey, J. (ed.), 'Brain facts: A primer on the brain and nervous system', 2nd edition, The Society for Neuroscience, Washington, DC, 1997.

3 Miranda, L., Schick, S., Dobson, C., Hogan, L. and B. D. Perry, 'Positive developmental effects of a brief music and movement program at a public pre-school', in press.

4 Miranda, L., Arthur, A., Milan, T., Mahoney, O. and B. D. Perry, 'The art of healing: The healing arts project, early childhood connections,' *Journal of Music and Movement Based Learning*, Vol. 4, pp. 35–40, 1998.

Chapter 6 Mastering the Senses

1 Carey, J. (ed.), 'Brain facts: A primer on the brain and nervous system', 2nd edition, The Society for Neuroscience, Washington, DC, 1997.

Chapter 7 From Curiosity to Learning

1 Greenspan, S. I., *The Growth of the Mind and the Endangered Origins of Intelligence*, Perseus Books, Massachusetts, 1997.

2 Perry, B. D., 'Memories of fear: How the brain stores and retrieves physiologic states, feelings, behaviours and thoughts from traumatic events,' *Images of the Body in Trauma*, Goodwin J. and R. Attias (eds.), Basic Books, New York, 1997.

Chapter 9 Sleeping and Dreaming

1 Carey, J. (ed.), 'Brain facts: A primer on the brain and nervous system', 2nd edition, The Society For Neuroscience, Washington, DC, 1997.

Chapter 10 When Things Go Wrong

1 Perry, B. D., 'Neurodevelopmental adaptations to violence: How children survive the intragenerational vortex of violence', *Violence and Childhood Trauma: Understanding and Responding to the Effects of Violence on Young Children*, Urban Child Research Center, Cleveland State University, 1996.

2 Perry, B. D., Pollard, R., Blakeley, T., Baker, W. and D. Vigilante, 'Childhood trauma, the neurobiology of adaptation and "use-dependent" development of the brain: How "states" become "traits,"' *Infant Mental Health*, Vol. 16, pp. 271–91, 1995.

3 Frater, S. and C. Waldegrave, 'Below the line: An analysis of income and poverty in New Zealand 1984–98,' The Family Centre, Lower Hutt, draft document discussed on Radio NZ, January, 2000.

4 Felitti, V. J., Anda, R. F., Nordenberg, D., Williamson, D. F., Spitz, A. M., Edwards, V., Koss, M. P. and J. S. Marks, 'Relationship of childhood abuse and household dysfunction to many of the leading causes of death in adults: the adverse childhood

experiences (ACE) study,' *American Journal of Preventive Medicine*, Vol. 14, pp. 245–58, 1998.

Chapter 11 Nutrition, the Brain and Health

1 Barker, D. J., 'Maternal nutrition, fetal nutrition, and disease in later life', *Nutrition*, Vol., 13, pp 807–13, 1997.

2 Guesry, P., 'The role of nutrition on brain development', *Preventive Medicine*, Vol. 27, pp. 189–94, 1998.

3 Morley, R. and A. Lucas, 'Nutrition and cognitive development', *British Medical Bulletin*, Vol. 53, pp. 123–34, 1997.

4 McEwen, B. S., 'Protective and damaging effects of stress mediators', *Seminars in Medicine of the Beth Israel Deaconess Medical Center*, Vol. 338, pp. 171–9, 1998.

Chapter 12 Personality and Temperament

1 Karr-Morse, R. and M. S. Wiley, *Ghosts From The Nursery: Tracing The Roots of Violence,* The Atlantic Monthly Press, New York, 1997.

Chapter 13 The Challenge

1 Cook, L. (ed.), 'New Zealand now: Children', Statistics New Zealand, Wellington, 1998.

2 Hertzman, C., 'Population health and human development', *Developmental Health and the Wealth of Nations,* Keating, D.P. and C. Hertzman, (eds.), Guilford Press, New York, 1999.

3 Hewlett, S.A., 'Child neglect in rich nations', UNICEF, New York, 1993.

4 Richardson, G., 'A welcome for every child: How France protects maternal and child health', National Center for Education in Maternal and Child Health, Arlington, VA, 1994.

5 McCain, M. and J. F. Mustard, (eds.), 'Reversing the real brain drain: Early years study report', Ontario Children's Secretariat, Toronto, 1999.

6 Principle of First Call, The World Summit on Children, New York, 1990.

BIBLIOGRAPHY AND FURTHER READING

Carey, J. (ed.) *'Brain facts: A primer on the brain and nervous system'*, third edition, Society for Neuroscience, Washington DC, 1997.

Connolly, K. J. and H. Forssberg, *Neurophysiology and Neuropsychology of Motor Development*, Mac Keith Press, London, 1997.

Gopnik, A., Meltzoff, A. N. and P. K. Kuhl, *The Scientist in The Crib: Minds, Brains, and How Children Learn*, William Morrow and Company Inc., New York, 1999.

Greenfield, S. S., *The Human Brain: A Guided Tour*, Weidenfield and Nicolson, London, 1997.

Greenspan, S. I. G., *The Growth of the Mind and the Endangered Origins of Intelligence,* Perseus Books, Massachusetts, 1997.

Hooper, J. and D. Teresi, *The 3-Pound Universe,* Macmillan, New York, 1996.

Karr-Morse, R. and M. S. Wiley, *Ghosts from the Nursery: Tracing the Roots of Violence*, The Atlantic Monthly Press, New York, 1997.

Kotulak, R., *Inside the Brain,* Andrews and McMeel, Kansas, 1996.

Nash, J. M., 'Fertile Minds', *Time*, 3 February, 1997.

Scott, T. and T. Grice, *The Great Brain Robbery*, The Publishing Trust, Wellington, 1996.

Shore, R. *Rethinking the Brain: New Insights into Early Development,* Families and Work Institute, New York, 1997.